# Heartburn Healing

## A Holistic Journey

------------

## Comprehensive Strategies For Acid Reflux & GERD Relief

**PLUS: Complete Guide to Medications**

"Dedicated to the readers embarking on this journey, may this book serve as a beacon of hope and a source of strength. It is my sincerest wish that within these pages, you find the guidance, inspiration, and comfort you are looking for. May it light your path to healing, understanding, and growth."

Lillian Heart ♡

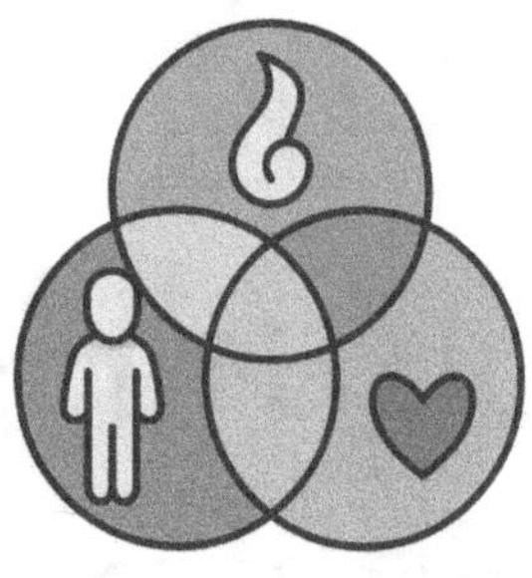

"This book provides medical information intended for educational purposes and should not be taken as professional medical advice or treatment. It is crucial to consult a healthcare provider for any medical concerns. Relying solely on the contents of this book for medical decisions is strongly discouraged. The author and publisher assume no responsibility for any adverse effects or consequences from the application of the information provided herein. Prioritize your health by always seeking professional guidance."

# Heartburn Healing
## A Holistic Journey

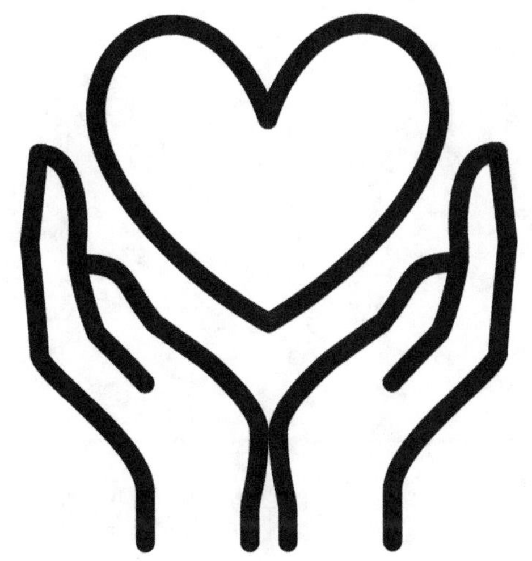

To Your Health

# Contents

# Strategies For Relief

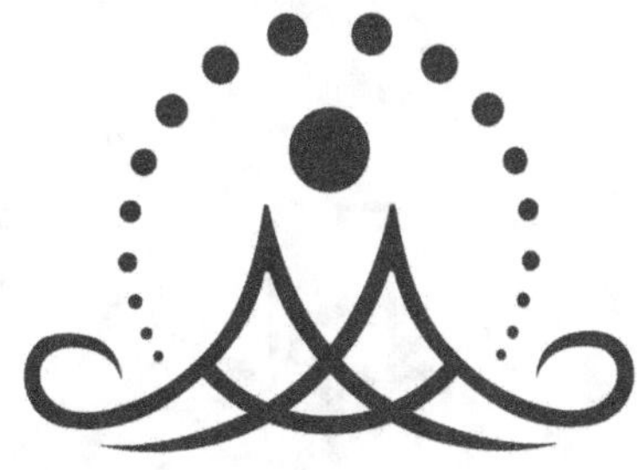

# Medical Remedies



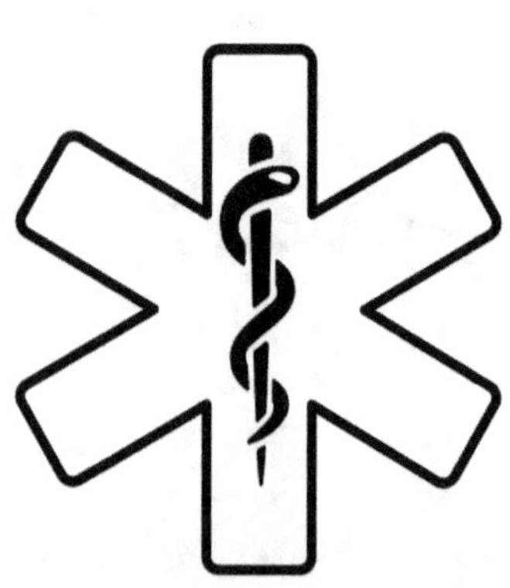

# Surgical Options



*Thank You* ♡

# Introduction

Get ready to embark on an exhilarating journey to reclaim your health and vitality! Imagine a life where the constant discomfort of heartburn doesn't dictate your choices, where your medicine cabinet or Doctor's prescription pad isn't your first stop for relief. Do you believe prevention is always better than a cure? Then this book is your roadmap to that reality. We're diving deep into a holistic healing adventure with one main goal: to free you from the clutches of medications, or at the very least, drastically cut down your dependence on them.

Armed with powerful strategies and easy-to-implement lifestyle changes, we're not just scratching the surface; we're going all in. From simple tweaks you can start today to more intricate plans requiring your dedication and commitment, we're on a mission to diminish, and possibly eliminate, your need for pharmaceuticals, avoiding the surgical route entirely.

But this isn't a book on exercise and dieting. No, this is a laser-focused guide designed to demystify the complex world of stomach acid and heartburn. We'll uncover the root causes of your discomfort, helping you sidestep those triggers once and for all.

Plus, we've compiled a comprehensive reference to almost every medication out there, transforming you into a savvy consumer, ready to navigate the overwhelming sea of choices in the pharmacy with confidence and clarity. I'm betting there will be a few surprises in store for you.

Rather than compiling a massive list of definitions every time a medical term or condition is mentioned, a thorough and complete '**Glossary of Terms**' with extended definitions is available at the end of this book for your reference and further exploration.

Therefore, if you encounter a word or term that isn't immediately understandable, feel free to pause and consult the glossary for clarification, it will most likely be there. Moreover, in the printed edition of this book, any term highlighted in *bold or italics* indicates its inclusion in the glossary, serving as a quick reference guide.

Prepare to be empowered, enlightened, and most importantly, relieved. This book isn't just about managing symptoms—it's about revolutionizing your approach to health. Say goodbye to guesswork and hello to a life of freedom and control. Your journey to wellness starts now.

Let's dive right in with some basics...

# ONE
## What is Heartburn/Acid Reflux?

*Heartburn*, characterized by a burning discomfort in the chest or throat, is known by a myriad of names, both in everyday language and medical jargon. The variety of terms reflects the different aspects and even severity associated with the condition.

To provide a foundational understanding, we will include a brief explanation of several of these terms that will be used throughout this book. This initial reference aims to clarify the terminology and ensure readers are well-informed about the various ways this widespread condition can be described and understood.

For example, *'Acid Reflux'* is often used interchangeably with heartburn, yet it specifically refers to the action of stomach acid flowing back into the *Esophagus*. In more severe cases, this condition is identified as *GERD*, or *Gastroesophageal Reflux Disease*, indicating a chronic pattern of reflux that can lead to more serious health issues.

Another related term, *'Indigestion,'* encompasses a broader range of gastrointestinal discomforts, including heartburn. Understanding these terms is important as they guide both diagnosis and treatment strategies, highlighting the importance of recognizing the differences and connections between these conditions.

Though certainly not a complete list, here are a few commonly used terms and brief definitions that are similar to or used in place of heartburn:

**Acid Reflux:** *Acid reflux* is a condition in which ***stomach acid*** flows back into the *esophagus*, the tube connecting the mouth and stomach. This backflow can cause irritation and a burning sensation in the chest, commonly referred to as heartburn.

**Gastroesophageal Reflux Disease (GERD):** *Gastroesophageal Reflux Disease (GERD)* is a chronic digestive disorder that occurs when stomach acid frequently flows back into the tube connecting the mouth and stomach (***Esophagus***). This acid reflux can irritate the lining of the esophagus, leading to symptoms like persistent heartburn, regurgitation of food or sour liquid, and difficulty swallowing. GERD is more severe and long-lasting than occasional acid reflux.

**Acid Indigestion:** *Acid indigestion*, also known as ***Dyspepsia***, is a term used to describe discomfort or pain in the upper abdomen often associated with eating. It is characterized by symptoms such as bloating, belching, nausea, and a feeling of fullness that is uncomfortable. While similar to heartburn, it encompasses a broader range of digestive symptoms and may not always involve acid reflux.

**Dyspepsia:** *Dyspepsia*, commonly referred to as indigestion, is a medical term describing a condition characterized by chronic or recurrent pain or discomfort in the upper abdomen. Symptoms often include bloating, nausea, belching, and a feeling of fullness after eating.

**Pyrosis:** *Pyrosis* is simply the medical term for what is commonly known as heartburn, often used in a clinical context. Typically occurring in the chest but may also extend to the neck, throat, or angle of the jaw.

**Sour Stomach:** Sour stomach, also known as acid stomach, indigestion, or upset stomach, refers to a range of gastrointestinal symptoms that can include heartburn, acid reflux, bloating, gas, and even nausea.

**Hyperacidity:** *Hyperacidity*, also known as acid dyspepsia, is a condition characterized by an excessive production of stomach acid.

**Gastric Reflux (GER):** Similar to *GERD*, gastric reflux involves the backward flow of stomach contents, including acid, into the esophagus.

# TWO

# Why Stomach Acid is Essential

## Protein Digestion

*Stomach Acid*, scientifically known as *Hydrochloric Acid (HCl)*, plays an indispensable role in the digestion of proteins, a crucial process for our nutritional health. When we consume protein-rich foods, they're not immediately usable by our bodies. They first need to be broken down into their building blocks—*Amino Acids*—and stomach acid is key to initiating this process.

Think of proteins as complex, folded structures, much like intricate origami. Stomach acid effectively "unfolds" these structures, exposing the bonds that hold the *amino acids* together. This unfolding, or *Denaturation*, is vital because it makes proteins more accessible to *Digestive Enzymes*. Without sufficient stomach acid, proteins remain in their complex forms and are much harder to break down, potentially leading to digestive issues and nutrient absorption problems.

Moreover, stomach acid activates an essential enzyme called *Pepsinogen*, converting it into *Pepsin*. *Pepsin* is the main enzyme responsible for breaking down proteins into smaller *Peptides*, which can then be further digested as they move through the *Gastrointestinal Tract*. This conversion from *pepsinogen* to *pepsin* wouldn't occur in a less acidic environment, highlighting the critical nature of stomach acid in protein digestion.

Finally, the presence of stomach acid triggers other digestive processes, including the release of hormones and digestive juices that facilitate the complete digestion and absorption of proteins.

In essence, stomach acid is foundational to our ability to digest proteins, ensuring that we can efficiently utilize these vital nutrients for bodily functions, muscle repair, and energy. As we delve deeper into the study of human biology and nutrition, the significance of such biochemical processes in maintaining health becomes increasingly apparent.

# Pathogen Defense

Stomach acid, predominantly *hydrochloric acid (HCl)*, is not just a crucial player in food digestion; it also serves as a formidable defender against **Pathogens** that enter our bodies through the food we consume. This acidic environment in the stomach acts as a gatekeeper, protecting us from various bacteria, viruses, and parasites that pose risks to our health.

When we think about the stomach, we often focus on its role in breaking down food. However, its acidic nature is equally important for *pathogen* defense. The stomach's acidity, with a pH ranging from 1.5 to 3.5, creates a hostile environment for most *pathogens*. This natural barrier effectively inactivates or kills many harmful *Microorganisms* before they can reach the intestines, where they might otherwise colonize and cause infections. It's fascinating to consider how this simple chemical barrier is our first line of defense in the *gastrointestinal tract.*

Moreover, the acidic environment helps to maintain the balance of **Gut Flora** by favoring the growth of beneficial **Bacteria** adapted to acidic conditions while inhibiting the growth of potential pathogens. This balance is crucial for gut health and, by extension, for the immune system, given the gut's significant role in immune function.

However, it's worth noting that not all *pathogens* are deterred by stomach acid. Some, like the bacteria **Helicobacter Pylori**, have adapted to survive and even thrive in acidic environments, leading to infections and conditions such as ulcers. This exception underscores the complexity of our bodies' interactions with microorganisms and the ongoing arms race between our defense mechanisms and pathogens.

Research into how stomach acid affects the **Microbiome** and *pathogen* defense is a vibrant field, shedding light on the intricate ways our bodies maintain health. As we continue to study these mechanisms, we gain a deeper appreciation for the sophisticated defense strategies our bodies employ, starting with something as seemingly simple as the acidic environment in our stomachs.

Understanding the protective role of stomach acid against pathogens enriches our knowledge of human physiology and underscores the importance of maintaining a healthy digestive system as part of overall health and well-being.

## Nutrient Absorption

Stomach acid is also crucial for the absorption of vital nutrients. This might seem a bit counterintuitive at first—how does something as corrosive as acid help in absorbing nutrients? Yet, the acidic environment of the stomach is essential for nutrient absorption, particularly for vitamins and minerals critical to our overall health.

First off, stomach acid facilitates the digestion of proteins, as mentioned earlier, by denaturing them and making them more accessible for enzymatic breakdown into *amino acids*. These *amino acids* are then absorbed in the intestines and are vital for numerous bodily functions, including tissue repair and growth. But the role of stomach acid doesn't stop there; it's also instrumental in the absorption of vitamin B12, an essential nutrient for nerve function and blood cell production. Vitamin B12 is bound to proteins in food, and stomach acid is necessary to release it, making it available for absorption later in the small intestine.

Moreover, the acidity in the stomach helps to solubilize minerals such as calcium, iron, and magnesium, transforming them into forms that can be more easily absorbed in the intestines. For instance, ***Non-Heme Iron***, found in plant sources, is converted into a more soluble form in the presence of stomach acid, enhancing its absorption. Similarly, calcium absorption is facilitated by stomach acid, playing a crucial role in bone health.

Interestingly, the acid also helps prevent the overgrowth of bacteria in the stomach and intestines, ensuring that the nutrients in the food we consume are available for our bodies to absorb, rather than being utilized by harmful bacteria.

However, conditions that reduce stomach acidity, such as chronic use of antacids or certain medical conditions, can lead to deficiencies in these nutrients. This highlights the delicate balance our bodies maintain and the essential role of stomach acid in our digestive health and overall well-being.

In understanding the multifaceted functions of stomach acid, it becomes clear that it's not just a substance for breaking down food but a critical component in the complex process of nutrient absorption, underscoring the interconnectedness of various bodily functions and the importance of maintaining a healthy digestive system.

# Activates Digestive Enzymes

Stomach acid plays an additional crucial role in our digestion process, especially when it comes to activating *digestive enzymes*. One key player is *pepsinogen*, which is the precursor to *pepsin*, the main enzyme responsible for breaking down proteins in our diet. Without the acidic environment provided by stomach acid, *pepsinogen* wouldn't convert to *pepsin*, making protein digestion inefficient.

This conversion is vital because it ensures that proteins are broken down into *peptides* and *amino acids*, which our bodies can then use for repair, growth, and energy. The acidity of the stomach also sets the stage for the optimal activity of these enzymes. Many digestive enzymes, including *pepsin*, require a specific acidic pH to function effectively. Without enough stomach acid, the digestive process slows down, leading to potential nutrient malabsorption and various digestive issues.

Moreover, stomach acid's role in enzyme activation highlights the body's clever mechanism to prevent self-digestion. By producing enzymes in their inactive forms, it safeguards the cells that produce them, activating these enzymes only when they're in the safe, acidic environment of the stomach.

# Prevents Bacterial Overgrowth

Stomach acid, predominantly *hydrochloric acid (HCl)*, plays a pivotal role in the body's defense mechanism against bacterial overgrowth, safeguarding our digestive system's health. This acidic environment within the stomach acts as a sterilizing agent, eliminating potentially harmful bacteria ingested with food and drink. Without this acidic barrier, our *gastrointestinal tract* would be vulnerable to colonization by **pathogenic bacteria**, leading to infections and a host of digestive disorders.

The importance of stomach acid in preventing bacterial overgrowth extends beyond just warding off acute infections. It is integral to maintaining the balance of the **Gut Microbiome**, the complex community of **Microorganisms** living in our digestive tract. An imbalance, or **Dysbiosis**, can result in conditions like small intestinal bacterial overgrowth (SIBO) and **Clostridium Difficile Infections**, which are associated with symptoms such as bloating, diarrhea, and abdominal pain.

Furthermore, adequate levels of stomach acid prevent the excessive proliferation of bacteria that could otherwise compete with the host for nutrients, potentially leading to nutritional deficiencies. It's this acid that ensures our gut environment remains balanced, supporting not just digestion but our overall health by protecting against bacterial overgrowth and its related complications.

In essence, stomach acid is not merely involved in food digestion; it's a critical component of our immune defense, keeping harmful bacteria at bay and preserving the health and integrity of our gastrointestinal ecosystem.

## Stimulates Hormone Secretion

Stomach acid, primarily composed of *hydrochloric acid (HCl)*, plays a multifaceted role in the digestive process, one of which includes the crucial task of stimulating hormone secretion. This function is pivotal for coordinating various aspects of digestion and ensuring the body efficiently utilizes the nutrients from the food we consume.

The presence of stomach acid triggers the release of **Gastrin**, a hormone produced by the stomach lining. *Gastrin* plays a key role in the digestive process by stimulating the gastric glands to produce more *hydrochloric acid*, creating a positive feedback loop that ensures enough acid is available to digest food properly. This mechanism highlights the body's ability to regulate digestive functions based on need, ensuring optimal conditions for food breakdown.

Additionally, the acidic environment in the stomach prompts the secretion of other hormones like **Secretin** and **Cholecystokinin (CCK)** from the small intestine. *Secretin* is released in response to the acidity of **Chyme** (partially digested food) entering the small intestine, signaling the **Pancreas** to release bicarbonate to neutralize the acid, protecting the intestinal lining and creating the right pH for enzyme activity. CCK, on the other hand, is released in response to fats and proteins in the *chyme*, and it stimulates the gallbladder to release **Bile**, aiding in fat digestion and absorption.

These hormones collectively orchestrate the digestive process, regulating the secretion of digestive juices, ensuring the proper breakdown and absorption of nutrients, and maintaining the overall health of the *gastrointestinal tract*. The stimulation of hormone secretion by stomach acid exemplifies the body's intricate regulation of digestion, emphasizing the essential role of stomach acid not just in breaking down food, but in facilitating a harmonious digestive process.

## Regulates GI Motility

Stomach acid, predominantly composed of *hydrochloric acid (HCl)*, is a vital player in the *gastrointestinal (GI)* system, going beyond its primary role in food digestion. An often overlooked yet critical function of stomach acid is its role in regulating **GI Motility**—the coordinated contraction and relaxation of muscles in the *gastrointestinal tract* that propels food through the digestive system. Understanding the significance of stomach acid in this context reveals its broader impact on digestive health and nutrient assimilation.

The process begins in the stomach, where the presence of acid not only breaks down food but also signals the readiness of the *chyme* (partially digested food and stomach acid mixture) to move into the small intestine. This acidic environment is essential for the activation of *pepsin* from its precursor, *pepsinogen*, facilitating protein digestion. However, stomach acid's influence extends to how it communicates with the small intestine, regulating the pace at which *chyme* is released. The release of *chyme* into the small intestine triggers the secretion of hormones like *secretin* and *cholecystokinin* (*CCK*), which play pivotal roles in digestion and also in modulating the motility of the **GI tract**.

*Secretin*, released in response to the acidity of *chyme*, has a dual function. It stimulates the *pancreas* to produce bicarbonate-rich pancreatic juice, neutralizing stomach acid, and it also acts on the stomach to regulate its emptying, ensuring that the small intestine can effectively process the *chyme* without being overwhelmed. Similarly, *CCK*, released in response to fats and proteins in the *chyme*, not only stimulates bile release from the gallbladder but also modulates gastric emptying and intestinal motility to optimize fat digestion and absorption.

Moreover, stomach acid influences the motility of the *GI tract* through its role in maintaining the microbial balance. By creating an acidic barrier, it prevents the overgrowth of pathogenic bacteria, ensuring that the *GI tract* operates smoothly without the interference of bacterial-induced disruptions in motility.

The regulation of *GI motility* by stomach acid is a testament to the body's intricate system of checks and balances. It ensures that each segment of the digestive process occurs timely and efficiently, allowing for optimal digestion, absorption of nutrients, and the smooth transit of waste materials. Insufficient stomach acid can lead to digestive imbalances, including slowed gastric emptying, altered intestinal transit times, and disruptions in the normal **Microbial Flora**, all of which can impact nutrient absorption and overall digestive health.

In summary, the role of stomach acid in regulating *GI motility* underscores its importance in the digestive system. It highlights the necessity of maintaining adequate levels of stomach acid not only for the breakdown and digestion of food but also for ensuring the coordinated movement of contents through the *GI tract*, contributing to the overall efficiency and effectiveness of digestive function.

# Supports Immune Function

Stomach acid plays a crucial role in supporting the body's immune function. Understanding the multifaceted contributions of stomach acid to our immune defense offers a fascinating insight into our body's complex mechanisms for maintaining health.

The stomach's acidic environment is one of the body's first lines of defense against ingested *pathogens*. Every day, we consume a vast array of bacteria, viruses, and other *microorganisms* through our food and drink. The potent acidity of stomach acid (with a pH ranging from 1.5 to 3.5) creates a hostile environment that neutralizes most of these potential invaders before they can enter the intestines and potentially cause infections. This protective barrier function is fundamental, as it prevents the colonization and proliferation of *pathogenic microorganisms* in the *gastrointestinal tract*, which could otherwise lead to illness and compromise immune function.

Moreover, the role of stomach acid in immune function extends to modulating the composition of the *Gut Microbiota*. The *gut microbiome*, comprising trillions of *microorganisms*, plays a crucial role in the development and function of the immune system. By regulating the survival of bacteria in the stomach and upper part of the small intestine, stomach acid helps maintain a balanced microbial ecosystem. This balance is vital for gut health and immunity, as a healthy microbiome stimulates the **Gut-Associated Lymphoid Tissue (GALT)**, a key component of the immune system, enhancing the body's overall immune responses.

Stomach acid also facilitates the absorption of critical nutrients that are essential for immune function. For example, it aids in the absorption of vitamin B12, zinc, and iron—nutrients that are crucial for the production and function of immune cells. Vitamin B12 deficiency, for instance, can lead to **Anemia** and weaken the body's ability to produce adequate immune responses. The acidic environment ensures these nutrients are ionized and more easily absorbed in the intestines, directly supporting the body's ability to maintain a robust immune system.

Furthermore, the acid-triggered conversion of *pepsinogen* to *pepsin* not only assists in protein digestion but indirectly supports immune function by ensuring the adequate breakdown of dietary proteins into *amino acids*. These *amino acids* are vital for synthesizing antibodies and other immune proteins, highlighting another link between stomach acid, nutrition, and immune health.

In essence, the importance of stomach acid transcends its digestive function, playing an indispensable role in supporting immune function. It acts as a gatekeeper, preventing *pathogen* entry, regulating the *gut microbiome,* and ensuring the absorption of nutrients critical for immune health. These insights underscore the delicate balance our bodies navigate to protect us from disease and maintain health.

As we progress in our exploration and comprehension of human biology, appreciating the interconnectedness of digestive health and immune function becomes crucial for fostering a **Holistic** view of human health and well-being. Recognizing the importance of maintaining optimal levels of stomach acid not only informs our approach to dietary and lifestyle choices but also highlights the potential impact of medical interventions that alter gastric acidity on our overall immune resilience.

## Facilitates Mineral Release

Stomach acid also serves a crucial function in facilitating the release of minerals from the foods we consume. It's amazing to uncover how this acidic environment is crucial for mineral absorption, a process vital for maintaining overall health.

Minerals such as calcium, magnesium, iron, and zinc are essential nutrients that support a wide range of bodily functions, from bone health to immune system operation. However, these minerals are often consumed in forms that are not readily available for absorption. This is where stomach acid comes into play. Its acidity helps to dissolve these minerals, transforming them into *Ionic*

*Forms* that the body can easily absorb. For instance, the acidic environment is particularly important for the absorption of iron, a mineral crucial for blood production. *Non-heme iron*, found in plant sources, requires the acidic conditions in the stomach to convert it into a soluble form that can be absorbed in the intestine.

Moreover, the release and subsequent absorption of minerals are not just about supporting structural functions and *Enzymatic Reactions*; they also play a role in nerve transmission, muscle function, and maintaining a healthy pH balance in the body. Without sufficient stomach acid, the efficiency of these processes could be compromised, leading to potential deficiencies despite adequate dietary intake.

In essence, the role of stomach acid is integral to ensuring that our bodies can utilize the essential minerals needed for optimal health and functioning. This highlights the interconnectedness of digestive health with overall well-being, underscoring the importance of maintaining a healthy balance of stomach acid.

## Summary

Stomach acid, primarily *hydrochloric acid (HCl)*, is a key player in our digestive health, serving multiple essential roles beyond just breaking down the food we eat. From optimizing nutrient absorption, to activating *digestive enzymes* like *pepsin* for protein breakdown to facilitating the release and absorption of vital minerals such as calcium and iron. Its low pH level not only aids in dissolving food but also acts as a barrier against harmful *pathogens*, protecting us from infections. Moreover, stomach acid is instrumental in stimulating hormone secretion that regulates digestion and *gut motility*, ensuring food moves correctly through our system.

Understanding the multifaceted importance of stomach acid underscores its significance in maintaining overall health, highlighting the intricate balance our bodies maintain to function optimally. This knowledge emphasizes the need to address issues like acid reflux not just for comfort but to preserve these critical digestive processes.

# THREE
# Dangers of Untreated Heartburn

Untreated heartburn, often dismissed as a common inconvenience, can pose substantial risks to both immediate comfort and long-term health. What may seem like a sporadic occurrence of discomfort can evolve into a chronic condition known as *gastroesophageal reflux disease (GERD)*, with implications that extend far beyond momentary inconvenience. The dangers of untreated heartburn encompass a spectrum of health issues, ranging from esophageal complications to respiratory problems, dental erosion, and even an increased risk of certain cancers.

One of the primary dangers associated with untreated heartburn is the development of **Esophagitis**. This condition involves inflammation of the esophagus due to the repeated exposure of its delicate lining to stomach acid. Persistent irritation can lead to erosions, ulcers, and potentially severe complications such as bleeding. In severe cases, untreated *esophagitis* may result in the formation of scar tissue, leading to a condition known as **Esophageal Stricture**. *Esophageal strictures* can cause difficulty swallowing, chest pain, and food impaction, significantly impacting an individual's quality of life.

As heartburn remains untreated, the chronic irritation and inflammation of the esophagus can lead to *Barrett's Esophagus*, a precancerous condition. *Barrett's esophagus* is characterized by a change in the cells lining the lower esophagus. Individuals with *Barrett's esophagus* face an increased risk of developing **Esophageal Adenocarcinoma**, a type of cancer that, if left undetected and untreated, can progress rapidly and have poor survival outcomes. Thus, untreated heartburn can evolve into a serious, potentially life-threatening condition with profound implications for long-term health.

Untreated heartburn can also manifest as respiratory complications. The regurgitation of stomach acid into the esophagus can trigger respiratory symptoms such as coughing, wheezing, and exacerbate pre-existing conditions like asthma. In some cases, the inhalation of gastric contents into the lungs can lead to **Aspiration Pneumonia**, a serious respiratory infection. The association between untreated heartburn and respiratory issues underscores the interconnected nature of the digestive and respiratory systems and highlights the importance of addressing heartburn promptly to safeguard overall health.

Furthermore, the acidic nature of stomach contents can have detrimental effects on dental health. Chronic exposure to stomach acid can erode tooth enamel, leading to dental problems such as cavities, tooth sensitivity, and even tooth loss over time. Dental issues resulting from untreated heartburn can compromise oral health, adding another dimension to the comprehensive impact of this condition on overall well-being.

In addition to esophageal, respiratory, and dental complications, untreated heartburn can influence an individual's nutritional status. The discomfort associated with chronic heartburn can lead to reduced appetite, avoidance of certain foods, and altered eating patterns. Over time, this may result in inadequate nutrient intake, contributing to nutritional deficiencies. Malnutrition, in turn, can affect various bodily functions and exacerbate existing health conditions.

In conclusion, untreated heartburn should not be underestimated. Its potential to progress into chronic conditions like *GERD, esophagitis, Barrett's esophagus,* and associated complications underscores the importance of early intervention. The interconnected nature of these risks, affecting the esophagus, respiratory system, dental health, and nutritional status, highlights the comprehensive impact of untreated heartburn on overall health.

Addressing the dangers of untreated heartburn necessitates a multifaceted approach, including, dietary changes, lifestyle modifications, and in some cases, medical interventions.

Risks more thoroughly explained:

## (GERD) Gastroesophageal Reflux Disease:

*Gastroesophageal Reflux Disease (GERD)*: is a chronic digestive disorder that occurs when stomach acid or, occasionally, *bile* flows back (refluxes) into the esophagus, the tube connecting the mouth and stomach. This backward flow can irritate the lining of the esophagus, leading to symptoms and potential complications. The primary symptom of *GERD* is heartburn. Other symptoms may include regurgitation of food or sour liquid, difficulty swallowing, coughing, wheezing, and chest pain, especially while lying down at night.

*GERD* is caused by frequent acid reflux—the action of stomach acid moving into the esophagus. A key player in this process is the *Lower Esophageal Sphincter (LES)*, a ring of muscle at the bottom of the esophagus. Normally, the *LES* closes as soon as food passes through it, but if the *LES* is weak or relaxes inappropriately, acid can flow back into the esophagus, causing *GERD* symptoms.

Factors that can contribute to *GERD* include obesity, pregnancy, smoking, eating large meals or lying down right after a meal, and consuming certain foods and drinks, such as alcohol, coffee, chocolate, fatty or spicy foods, and certain medications.

Management and treatment of *GERD* aim to reduce symptoms, heal the esophageal lining, and prevent complications. Lifestyle changes, such as weight loss, dietary adjustments, and avoiding triggers, play a crucial role. Medications may include **Antacids, H2 Receptor Blockers**, and **Proton Pump Inhibitors (PPIs)** to reduce acid production. In severe cases, surgical options like **Fundoplication** may be considered to strengthen the *LES* and prevent reflux. These will all be explained later in much greater detail.

*GERD* not only affects quality of life but can also lead to serious health issues, including *esophagitis, esophageal strictures*, and an increased risk of esophageal cancer, emphasizing the importance of management and treatment.

## Laryngopharyngeal Reflux (LPR):

*Laryngopharyngeal Reflux (LPR)*, also known as *Silent Reflux*, is a variant of *gastroesophageal reflux disease (GERD)* but with distinct characteristics and manifestations. Unlike *GERD*, which primarily affects the esophagus and is often marked by heartburn, *LPR* occurs when the stomach's contents, including acid and enzymes such as *pepsin*, travel back up beyond the esophagus into the larynx (voice box) and pharynx (throat), and sometimes even into the **Nasopharynx**, the part of the throat that connects to the nasal passages. This reflux can cause irritation and damage to these areas, leading to a variety of symptoms that are often unrelated to the typical symptoms associated with acid reflux.

The symptoms of *LPR* are diverse and can be misleading, often leading to misdiagnosis. Patients may experience chronic cough, hoarseness, a sensation of a lump in the throat (**Globus Pharyngeus**), difficulty swallowing (**Dysphagia**), frequent throat clearing, sore throat, and even changes in voice quality. Some may also experience breathing difficulties or a feeling of tightness in the throat. These symptoms arise because the larynx and throat are not equipped to handle the acidic and enzymatic content that refluxes from the stomach, making them more susceptible to irritation and inflammation.

The diagnosis of *LPR* is complex and typically involves a detailed patient history, physical examination, and specialized tests. One common diagnostic tool is **Laryngoscopy**, where a doctor uses a scope to view the throat and **Larynx** directly to look for signs of inflammation and damage. Another diagnostic method is pH monitoring, which measures the acidity level in the throat over a 24-hour period to confirm the presence of acid reflux.

The pathophysiology of *LPR* involves the dysfunction of both the **Lower Esophageal Sphincter (LES)**, which separates the stomach from the esophagus, and the

*Upper Esophageal Sphincter (UES)*, which protects the upper airway. When these sphincters fail to function properly, it allows the stomach contents to travel back up into the esophagus and potentially into the throat and *larynx.*

Treatment for *LPR* often involves a combination of lifestyle modifications, dietary changes, and medication. Lifestyle modifications may include weight loss, quitting smoking, and elevating the head of the bed to prevent reflux during sleep. Dietary changes typically involve avoiding foods and beverages that can trigger reflux, such as spicy foods, caffeine, alcohol, and chocolate. *Proton pump inhibitors (PPIs)* and *H2 blockers* are commonly prescribed medications that reduce stomach acid production, helping to alleviate symptoms and prevent further damage to the throat and *larynx.*

In more severe cases, or when conservative treatments fail to provide relief, surgery may be considered. Procedures such as *fundoplication* can help strengthen the *LES*, preventing reflux.

It is essential for individuals experiencing symptoms suggestive of *LPR* to seek medical evaluation and treatment. Left untreated, *LPR* can lead to chronic throat irritation, inflammation, and even significant damage to the vocal cords and respiratory system, affecting the quality of life. With appropriate diagnosis and management, most patients can achieve significant symptom relief and prevent long-term complications associated with *LPR*.

**Esophagitis:** *Esophagitis* is an inflammation of the *esophagus*, the muscular tube that transports food and liquids from the mouth to the stomach. This condition is characterized by several uncomfortable symptoms, including difficulty swallowing (**Dysphagia**), pain when swallowing (**Odynophagia**), chest pain, and a sensation of food stuck in the throat. The inflammation can damage the esophageal lining, leading to complications if left untreated.

The most common cause of *esophagitis* is *acid reflux*, also known as *gastroesophageal reflux disease (GERD)*, where stomach acid backs up into the *esophagus*, irritating its lining. However, *esophagitis* can also result from other factors, such as infections (especially in people with weakened immune systems), medications that can irritate the *esophagus* if not swallowed properly, and allergic reactions, such as **Eosinophilic Esophagitis**, where a type of white blood cell (**Eosinophil**) builds up in the lining of the esophagus in response to an allergen, causing inflammation.

Diagnosis of *esophagitis* typically involves **Endoscopy**, a procedure where a flexible tube with a light and camera (**Endoscope**) is inserted down the throat to examine the *esophagus* and, if necessary, to take a biopsy for further examination. Other tests might include *Barium Swallow Studies*, where X-rays are taken after the patient drinks a *barium* solution that coats the *esophagus*, highlighting abnormalities, or *Esophageal Manometry* to measure the rhythmic muscle contractions of the *esophagus* when swallowing.

Treatment for *esophagitis* depends on the underlying cause. For reflux-induced *esophagitis*, lifestyle modifications such as dietary changes, weight loss, and avoiding certain foods and drinks can be effective, alongside medications to reduce stomach acid and promote healing. Antiviral or antifungal medications can treat infectious *esophagitis*, while avoidance of known allergens and **Corticosteroids** are used for *Eosinophilic Esophagitis*.

If not properly managed, *esophagitis* can lead to complications like scarring, narrowing of the *esophagus* (strictures), or *Barrett's Esophagus*, a condition where the tissue lining the *esophagus* changes, increasing the risk of developing esophageal cancer. Therefore, early diagnosis and treatment are crucial to prevent long-term damage and ensure the health of the esophageal tissue.

**Esophageal Strictures:** *Esophageal Strictures* refer to the narrowing of the *esophagus*, the tube that carries food and liquids from the mouth to the stomach. This condition can significantly interfere with the passage of food and drink, leading to symptoms such as difficulty swallowing (*dysphagia*), regurgitation of food, weight loss, and a sensation of food being stuck in the chest. Strictures are often a complication of long-term irritation and damage to the esophageal lining, commonly resulting from chronic acid reflux or *(GERD)*. Other causes can include radiation therapy to the chest, ingestion of caustic substances, or surgical procedures involving the *esophagus*.

Diagnosis of *esophageal strictures* typically involves an *endoscopic* examination, where a thin, flexible tube with a camera (*endoscope*) is inserted through the mouth to view the *esophagus*. A *barium swallow study*, an X-ray test where the patient drinks a barium solution to provide clear imaging of the *esophagus*, can also be used.

Treatment aims to relieve symptoms and improve the passage of food. It often involves the dilation of the *esophagus*, where balloons or dilators are used to stretch and widen the narrowed area. Medications to treat the underlying cause of *acid reflux* and prevent further damage are also common. In severe cases, surgical intervention may be necessary to remove the stricture or reconstruct the affected area of the *esophagus*. Managing *esophageal strictures* effectively is crucial to maintain proper nutrition and quality of life.

**Barrett's Esophagus:** *Barrett's Esophagus* is a condition characterized by an abnormal change in the cells of the lower *esophagus*, a direct consequence of chronic inflammation due to acid reflux from the stomach or *gastroesophageal reflux disease (GERD)*. In *Barrett's Esophagus*, the normal esophageal lining (**Squamous Epithelium**) is replaced with a type of intestinal lining (**Columnar Epithelium**), which is more resistant to stomach acid but also more prone to developing *Esophageal Adenocarcinoma*, a type of cancer.

This condition is significant because it increases the risk of developing esophageal cancer, although the overall risk remains low. Patients with *Barrett's Esophagus* often do not exhibit symptoms beyond those associated with *GERD*, such as chronic heartburn, acid reflux, and difficulty swallowing. The diagnosis of *Barrett's Esophagus* typically requires an upper *gastrointestinal (GI) endoscopy* with biopsies. During this procedure, a **Gastroenterologist** examines the *esophagus* with a camera on a flexible tube inserted through the mouth and collects tissue samples to identify cellular changes indicative of *Barrett's Esophagus*.

The management of *Barrett's Esophagus* focuses on controlling acid reflux symptoms and monitoring the esophagus for early signs of progression towards cancer. Treatment options include lifestyle modifications, such as dietary changes, weight loss, and avoiding tobacco and alcohol, which can exacerbate acid reflux. Medications like *proton pump inhibitors (PPIs)* are frequently prescribed to reduce stomach acid and promote healing of the esophagus. In some cases, *endoscopic* procedures or surgery may be recommended to remove dysplastic (precancerous) cells or to treat early esophageal cancer.

Surveillance is a key component of managing *Barrett's Esophagus*. Regular **Endoscopic Exams** with **biopsies** are recommended to monitor the condition and detect any changes early. The frequency of these exams depends on the presence and severity of dysplasia found in biopsy samples.

Advancements in *endoscopic* treatments, such as **Radiofrequency Ablation (RFA)** and **Endoscopic Mucosal Resection (EMR)**, have shown promise in treating *dysplasia* and early cancer in patients with *Barrett's Esophagus*. These minimally invasive procedures target and remove or destroy abnormal cells while preserving the healthy esophageal tissue.

In summary, *Barrett's Esophagus* is a condition requiring careful monitoring and management due to its association with an increased risk of *esophageal cancer*. With appropriate treatment and surveillance, individuals with Barrett's Esophagus can manage their condition and significantly reduce their risk of developing advanced cancer.

**Esophageal Cancer:** *Esophageal Cancer* is a serious and potentially fatal condition that occurs in the *esophagus*, the long, hollow tube connecting the throat to the stomach. This type of cancer can emerge anywhere along the esophagus and is classified into two main types: ***Squamous Cell Carcinoma*** and ***Adenocarcinoma***. *Squamous cell carcinoma* originates in the *squamous cells* lining the esophagus and is more prevalent in the upper and middle parts of the esophagus. *Adenocarcinoma*, on the other hand, typically develops in the lower esophagus, arising from ***Glandular Cells*** that are often the result of changes due to conditions like *Barrett's Esophagus*, which is linked to chronic acid reflux or *GERD*.

Risk factors for esophageal cancer include smoking, heavy alcohol consumption, chronic acid reflux, obesity, a diet low in fruits and vegetables, and certain genetic conditions. The symptoms of *esophageal cancer* tend to appear once the disease has advanced and may include difficulty swallowing (*dysphagia*), weight loss, chest pain, worsening indigestion or heartburn, and coughing or hoarseness.

Diagnosis of *esophageal cancer* often involves a combination of *endoscopy*, where a flexible tube with a camera is used to examine the esophagus, and *biopsies*, where tissue samples are taken for analysis. Imaging tests, such as **CT Scans** and **PET Scans**, can help determine the extent (stage) of the cancer.

Treatment for *esophageal cancer* depends on the cancer's stage, location, and the patient's overall health. Options may include surgery to remove the tumor or part of the esophagus, **Chemotherapy**, **Radiation Therapy**, or a combination of these treatments. **Targeted Therapy** and **Immunotherapy** are newer treatments that may be options for certain patients.

Despite advances in treatment, *esophageal cancer* often has a poor prognosis because it is frequently diagnosed at an advanced stage. Early detection and treatment are critical for improving survival rates. Lifestyle changes to reduce the risk of acid reflux and *GERD*, such as maintaining a healthy weight, eating a balanced diet, and avoiding tobacco and excessive alcohol, can also help lower the risk of developing *esophageal cancer*.

**Asthma Exacerbations:** *Asthma Exacerbations*, or asthma attacks, can be significantly influenced by acid reflux (also known as GERD). This backward flow of acid can also affect the airways and lungs, potentially triggering or worsening asthma symptoms.

The relationship between asthma and acid reflux is complex and bidirectional. Acid reflux can provoke *asthma exacerbations* by causing direct irritation of the airways or through a reflex mechanism that leads to **Bronchoconstriction**, the narrowing of the air passages in the lungs. Conversely, asthma and the medications used to treat it can exacerbate *GERD* symptoms by increasing pressure changes in the chest and abdomen, which in turn can promote the reflux of acid into the *esophagus*.

Individuals with asthma who experience frequent exacerbations may find that managing their acid reflux can lead to better control of their asthma. Strategies to manage *GERD* include dietary changes, such as avoiding foods and drinks that trigger reflux (e.g., spicy foods, caffeine, alcohol), eating smaller meals, not lying down immediately after eating, and elevating the head of the bed. In some cases, medications like *proton pump inhibitors (PPIs)* or *H2 receptor antagonists* may be prescribed to reduce stomach acid production and alleviate reflux symptoms.

Understanding and addressing the connection between acid reflux and asthma is crucial for individuals affected by both conditions. By managing *GERD* effectively, it may be possible to reduce the frequency and severity of *asthma exacerbations*.

**Esophageal Ulcers:** *Esophageal Ulcers* are open sores or lesions that form on the lining of the *esophagus*, the tube that carries food from the mouth to the stomach. These ulcers result from damage to the esophageal lining, typically caused by the acidic digestive juices produced by the stomach. When stomach acid frequently backs up into the esophagus *(GERD)*, it can erode the esophageal lining and lead to the development of ulcers.

The symptoms of *esophageal ulcers* include severe, burning chest pain that can mimic heartburn, difficulty swallowing *(dysphagia)*, pain when swallowing *(odynophagia)*, nausea, and sometimes vomiting blood or passing black, **Tarry Stools**, indicating bleeding within the *esophagus*. These symptoms not only cause significant discomfort but can also interfere with nutritional intake and quality of life.

The diagnosis of *esophageal ulcers* typically involves *endoscopy*, a procedure in which a flexible tube with a light and camera *(endoscope)* is inserted through the mouth to visually inspect the *esophagus*. During *endoscopy*, a doctor can also take small tissue samples **(biopsy)** to test for infections, like those caused by the **Helicobacter Pylori Bacterium**, which can contribute to ulcer formation.

Treatment for *esophageal ulcers* focuses on reducing the factors that cause the ulcers, such as managing *GERD* or treating any underlying infections. Medications like *proton pump inhibitors (PPIs)* and *H2 receptor antagonists* are commonly prescribed to decrease stomach acid production, helping to heal the ulcer and relieve symptoms. In addition to medication, lifestyle changes, such as avoiding foods and beverages that trigger acid reflux, eating smaller meals, quitting smoking, and losing weight if overweight, are recommended to help manage the condition.

In severe cases, where ulcers lead to complications like significant bleeding or perforation of the *esophagus*, more intensive treatments or surgery may be required. Addressing *esophageal ulcers* promptly and effectively is crucial to prevent complications, alleviate symptoms, and promote healing of the esophageal lining.

**Aspiration Pneumonia:** *Aspiration Pneumonia* relating to acid reflux, *(GERD)*, occurs when the contents of the stomach, including highly acidic digestive juices, are inhaled into the lungs. This type of *aspiration pneumonia* is particularly concerning because the aspirated material is not only foreign to the lungs but also corrosive, leading to inflammation, infection, and damage to the lung tissues.

Acid reflux increases the risk of *aspiration pneumonia* by promoting the backward flow of stomach contents into the *esophagus* and potentially into the throat and respiratory tract, especially during sleep or in individuals with weakened esophageal or throat muscles. The risk is further heightened in those with conditions that impair consciousness or swallowing, such as neurological disorders, sleep apnea, or the use of sedatives or alcohol.

Symptoms of *aspiration pneumonia* induced by acid reflux may include persistent cough, chest pain, fever, shortness of breath, wheezing, and a worsening of pre-existing respiratory conditions. These symptoms arise from the body's response to the acidic material in the lungs, leading to an inflammatory reaction that can invite bacterial infection on top of the chemical injury caused by the acid.

Diagnosis involves a clinical assessment that may include a history of *GERD* symptoms, imaging studies like chest X-rays or *CT scans* to identify inflammation or infection in the lungs, and possibly a bronchoscopy to directly visualize and sample the lower airways.

Treatment typically focuses on addressing the underlying acid reflux with medications such as *proton pump inhibitors (PPIs)* or *H2 receptor antagonists* to reduce stomach acid production and prevent further aspiration. Antibiotics may be prescribed if a bacterial infection is present or suspected. Supportive care, including **Oxygen Therapy** and possibly **Bronchial Hygiene Techniques**, helps manage symptoms and promote lung healing.

Preventive measures are crucial for individuals with *GERD* to reduce the risk of *aspiration pneumonia*. These may include lifestyle and dietary changes to manage reflux, elevating the head of the bed, and avoiding eating or drinking close to bedtime. For those at high risk, careful monitoring and management of *GERD* are essential to prevent the potentially serious complications associated with *aspiration pneumonia*.

**Chronic Cough or Laryngitis:** *Chronic Cough* or *Laryngitis* in the context of acid reflux, is a manifestation of the irritation and inflammation caused by stomach acid and enzymes reaching the *larynx* (voice box) and throat. This condition, often termed *Laryngopharyngeal Reflux (LPR)*, occurs when the *lower esophageal sphincter (LES)* fails to function properly, allowing acid to escape the stomach and move upwards. Unlike traditional *GERD*, which primarily affects the *esophagus* and is characterized by heartburn, *LPR* can occur without heartburn, making the diagnosis less straightforward.

Acid reflux can lead to *chronic cough* and *laryngitis* due to the irritation of the voice box and respiratory tract. Individuals may experience a persistent cough that does not respond to typical cough remedies, hoarseness, a sensation of a lump in the throat, difficulty swallowing, or a constant need to clear the throat. These symptoms result from the delicate tissues of the throat and *larynx* being exposed to acidic contents, causing swelling, inflammation, and damage over time.

Diagnosing GERD-related chronic cough or *laryngitis* typically involves a detailed medical history, examination of the throat and *larynx*, possibly using **Laryngoscopy**, and may include pH monitoring to measure acid levels in the throat. Treatment strategies aim to reduce acid exposure to the *larynx* and throat, manage symptoms, and prevent further damage. This may include dietary and lifestyle modifications, such as avoiding foods that trigger reflux, eating smaller meals, and not lying down immediately after eating. Medications that reduce acid production, like *proton pump inhibitors*, are commonly prescribed. In some cases, surgery may be considered to strengthen the lower *esophageal sphincter*.

Effective management of acid reflux is crucial in treating chronic cough or *laryngitis* caused by *GERD*. By addressing the root cause and taking steps to minimize acid reflux, individuals can significantly reduce their symptoms and improve their quality of life. It's also important for patients to be aware of the potential for *GERD* to cause these symptoms, as they are often overlooked or misattributed to other conditions.

**Dental Problems:** Dental problems associated with acid reflux, *(GERD)*, stem from the damaging effects of stomach acid on **Tooth Enamel**. When acid from the stomach makes its way into the mouth, it can lead to erosion of the enamel, the hard, outer layer of the teeth. This erosion weakens teeth, making them more susceptible to decay, sensitivity, and discoloration.

Patients with *GERD* often experience increased tooth sensitivity, especially to hot, cold, or sweet foods and drinks. They may also notice their teeth becoming more translucent, brittle, and prone to chipping or cracking.

Additionally, acid reflux can contribute to bad breath and gum inflammation or disease due to the acidic environment altering the **Oral Microbiome**. Preventing these dental issues involves managing *GERD* through dietary changes, medications, and lifestyle adjustments, alongside maintaining rigorous oral hygiene and using fluoride treatments to strengthen tooth enamel. Regular dental check-ups are crucial for monitoring the health of the teeth and gums and addressing any problems early.

# FOUR
## Several Likely Causes

We've covered the basics of stomach acid and how heartburn arises when *hydrochloric acid* backs up into the *esophagus*, causing irritation and a burning feeling. We've also touched on its critical role in digestion and the potential risks if it's not managed properly. Aging, beyond our control, makes acid reflux more common, but it's crucial to remember that experiences with heartburn vary from person to person.

When we look into the standard triggers, it becomes clear that while preventing heartburn isn't always possible, there are numerous ways to manage and alleviate its symptoms even with the smallest of behavioral and lifestyle changes.

This understanding enables us to take significant steps toward minimizing discomfort and protecting our digestive health.

## Relaxation of the Lower Esophageal Sphincter (LES):

*The Lower Esophageal Sphincter (LES)* plays a pivotal role in digestive health, acting as a vital barrier between the stomach and the *esophagus*. Its primary function is to prevent the backflow of gastric contents into the esophagus. However, when the *LES* relaxes inappropriately or becomes weak, it fails to fulfill this crucial role effectively. This malfunction allows acidic and enzymatic contents from the stomach to flow back into the esophagus, leading to the discomfort and pain known as heartburn, acid reflux, *GERD* etc.

The inappropriate relaxation or weakening of the LES is at the core of many digestive problems. Persistent heartburn resulting from such reflux can cause significant irritation and inflammation of the esophageal lining. This chronic exposure to stomach acids and enzymes can lead to severe complications over time, including all the issues mentioned previously in chapter 3 "Dangers of Untreated heartburn". Including *esophagitis*, an inflamed esophagus; *Barrett's Esophagus*, where the esophageal lining changes; and even *esophageal cancer*, highlighting the importance of LES integrity for digestive wellness.

Addressing factors that contribute to the dysfunction of the LES, including dietary choices, lifestyle habits, and the use of certain medications, is essential in managing and preventing the onset of heartburn and more serious GERD-related conditions. Thus, maintaining the health and proper functioning of the LES is key to avoiding a broad spectrum of gastrointestinal issues, underscoring the importance of dietary and lifestyle modifications in promoting digestive health.

**Improper Function of the (UES):** *The Upper Esophageal Sphincter (UES)* and the *Lower Esophageal Sphincter (LES)* work in tandem to facilitate proper digestion and protect the *esophagus* from damage. The UES, located at the top of the esophagus, controls the passage of food and air into the esophagus from the throat, while the LES, situated at the lower end, regulates the entry of food into the stomach and prevents gastric acid from flowing back into the esophagus.

When swallowing occurs, the UES relaxes to allow food or liquid to enter the esophagus. As the ***Bolus*** moves down, the muscular walls of the esophagus contract in a coordinated manner (***Peristalsis***) to propel it toward the stomach. Upon reaching the lower end, the LES relaxes at the right moment to permit the food to pass into the stomach. Immediately after, the LES contracts again to form a tight seal, preventing stomach contents, which are highly acidic, from refluxing into the esophagus, thereby protecting the esophageal lining from acid-induced damage.

The synchronized action between the UES and LES is crucial for maintaining the one-way movement of food and for safeguarding the esophagus against *GERD*. Disruptions in their function can lead to many digestive disorders, highlighting the importance of their harmonious operation in digestive health.

# Hiatal Hernia

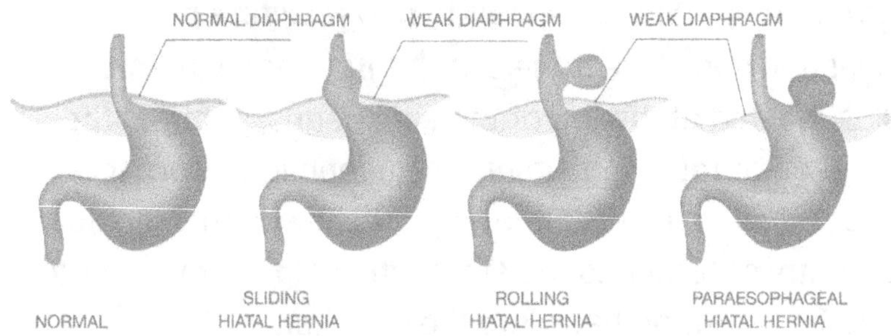


*Hiatal Hernias* allow stomach acid to flow back into the *esophagus*, causing heartburn and other symptoms. A condition where part of the stomach protrudes through the diaphragm into the chest cavity. There are two main types of *hiatal hernias*, each characterized by the nature and extent of stomach displacement:

A **Sliding Hiatal Hernia** is the most common type, where the **Gastroesophageal Junction** and a portion of the stomach slide upward into the chest cavity when a person is upright and move back into the abdominal cavity when lying down. This type is often associated with *gastroesophageal reflux disease (GERD)*.

A **Paraesophageal** or **Rolling Hiatal Hernia** involves the stomach protruding alongside the *esophagus* into the chest through the diaphragm. Unlike *sliding hernias*, the *gastroesophageal junction* remains in place. This type may cause severe symptoms like chest pain and difficulty swallowing. Complications, such as **Stomach**

*Strangulation* or obstruction, can occur, necessitating prompt medical attention.

It's important to note that not all *hiatal hernias* cause symptoms, and their presence may be incidental. Diagnosis and management often involve lifestyle modifications, medications to manage reflux, and, in severe cases, surgical intervention to repair the hernia and prevent complications. Individuals experiencing symptoms suggestive of *hiatal hernia* should seek medical evaluation for proper diagnosis and treatment.

## Delayed Stomach Emptying (Gastroparesis):

*Delayed stomach emptying*, or *Gastroparesis*, is a condition characterized by impaired or slowed movement of food from the stomach into the small intestine. This delay in gastric emptying disrupts the normal digestive process, leading to various symptoms and potential complications. The primary cause of *gastroparesis* is often dysfunction of the *Vagus Nerve*, a crucial component of the digestive system responsible for controlling the muscles of the stomach.

### <u>Causes:</u>

The most common cause of *gastroparesis* is damage to the *vagus nerve*. This damage can result from various factors, including:

- Diabetes: Prolonged high blood sugar levels in diabetes can lead to nerve damage, affecting the vagus nerve.
- Post-Surgical Complications: Surgeries on the stomach or vagus nerve can contribute to gastroparesis.
- Certain Medications: Some medications, particularly those that affect the nervous system, can interfere with stomach contractions.
- Viral Infections: Infections affecting the stomach muscles or nerves can cause gastroparesis.
- Neurological Conditions: Conditions such as Parkinson's disease and multiple sclerosis can impact nerve function, including the *vagus nerve*.

## *Symptoms:*

The symptoms of *gastroparesis* can vary in severity and may include:

- Nausea and Vomiting: Persistent nausea is a common symptom, and vomiting may occur, especially after eating.
- Feeling Full Quickly: Individuals with *gastroparesis* may experience early satiety, feeling excessively full even after consuming a small amount of food.
- Abdominal Discomfort: Bloating and abdominal discomfort are prevalent symptoms.

- Heartburn or Acid Reflux: Delayed stomach emptying can contribute to the reflux of stomach contents into the esophagus.
- Changes in Blood Sugar Levels: For individuals with diabetes, *gastroparesis* can lead to unpredictable blood sugar levels.

## Complications:

*Gastroparesis* can result in several complications, including:

- Malnutrition: Inadequate nutrient absorption due to delayed stomach emptying can lead to malnutrition.
- Dehydration: Difficulty in consuming enough fluids can result in dehydration.
- Bacterial Overgrowth: Slow transit can encourage bacterial overgrowth in the stomach, contributing to further digestive issues.
- Impaired Blood Sugar Control: *Gastroparesis* can make blood sugar control more challenging for individuals with diabetes.

## Diagnosis and Treatment:

Diagnosis involves a combination of medical history, physical examination, and diagnostic tests, including gastric emptying studies and imaging. Treatment aims to manage symptoms and may include:

- Dietary Modifications: Eating smaller, more frequent meals and avoiding certain foods.
- Medications: *Prokinetic Medications* to stimulate stomach contractions or antiemetics to control nausea.
- Surgical Interventions: In severe cases, surgery may be considered.

## <u>Lifestyle Management:</u>

- Eating smaller, more frequent meals.
- Chewing food thoroughly.
- Staying hydrated with fluids between meals.
- Avoiding high-fiber or high-fat foods.

*Gastroparesis* is a chronic condition that requires ongoing management. Individuals experiencing symptoms should seek medical evaluation for an accurate diagnosis and appropriate treatment plan tailored to their specific needs.

# Pregnancy

Pregnancy commonly leads to heartburn due to hormonal and physical changes that affect the digestive system. As the pregnancy hormone **Progesterone** increases, it relaxes the smooth muscles throughout the body, including the *lower esophageal sphincter (LES)*. When relaxed, it becomes less effective in preventing stomach acid from flowing back into the *esophagus*, leading to heartburn.

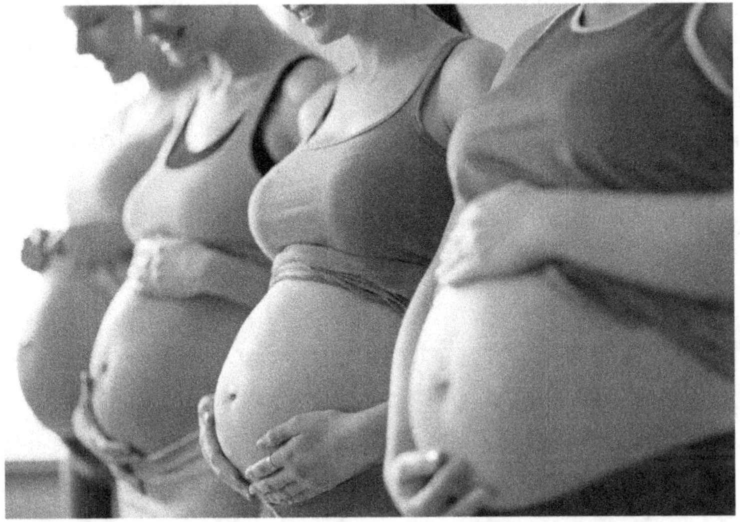

Additionally, the growing uterus exerts pressure on the stomach, pushing its contents upward. This pressure, combined with the hormonal influence on the *LES*, contributes to the reflux of stomach acid. As the pregnancy progresses, the expanding uterus further displaces abdominal organs, exacerbating the likelihood of heartburn.

Moreover, pregnant women may experience changes in eating habits, such as consuming smaller, more frequent meals, which can impact the stomach's digestive processes. Elevated levels of the hormone *Relaxin* also contribute to the relaxation of various muscles, potentially affecting the normal functioning of the digestive tract.

Alleviating heartburn during pregnancy involves lifestyle and dietary adjustments. Eating smaller, more frequent meals can reduce stomach pressure, and avoiding spicy, acidic, or fatty foods helps prevent acid reflux. Staying upright for at least an hour after eating and avoiding late meals before bedtime can also minimize symptoms. Elevating the head while sleeping creates a gravity-assisted barrier against stomach acid rising.

Additionally, drinking water between meals rather than with them can aid digestion without increasing stomach volume. Wearing loose-fitting clothing avoids putting extra pressure on the abdomen. If lifestyle changes are insufficient, it's important to consult a healthcare provider before taking any medications, as they can recommend safe treatments tailored to pregnancy-related heartburn.

# Obesity

**Being overweight can significantly contribute to the worsening and more frequent episodes of heartburn.**

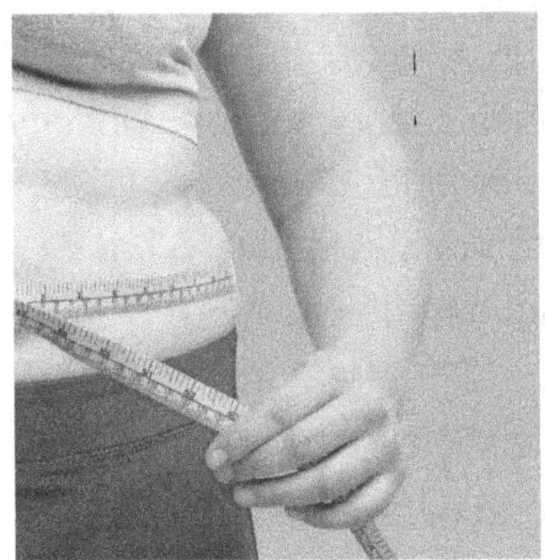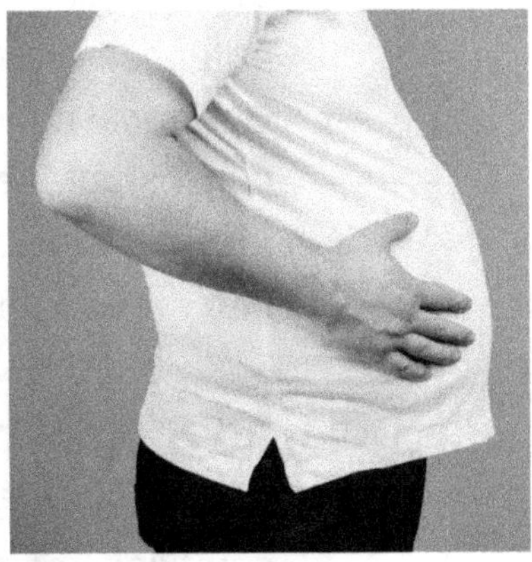

Several interconnected factors include:

## Increased Abdominal Pressure:

- *Obesity*, especially excess weight around the abdomen, leads to increased abdominal pressure. This added pressure can cause the *lower esophageal sphincter (LES)*, to weaken or become compromised.
- A weakened *LES* is less effective in preventing the backflow of stomach acid into the *esophagus*, promoting the occurrence of acid reflux and heartburn.

## Changes in Hormones:

- *Adipose Tissue*, or fat cells, produces hormones, some of which may influence the *LES*. **Leptin**, a hormone associated with appetite regulation and metabolism, has been implicated in relaxing the *LES* and potentially contributing to reflux.
- Hormonal changes associated with obesity can disrupt the normal functioning of the *LES*, allowing stomach acid to flow back into the esophagus more easily.

## Delayed Stomach Emptying:

- Obesity is linked to delayed stomach emptying, meaning that the stomach takes longer to empty its contents into the small intestine. This delayed transit allows stomach acid to remain in the stomach for an extended period, increasing the likelihood of reflux.
- Prolonged contact between stomach acid and the *esophagus* can lead to irritation, inflammation, and the characteristic symptoms of heartburn.

## Hiatal Hernia:

- Obesity is a known risk factor for *hiatal hernia*, a condition where a portion of the stomach protrudes into the chest through the diaphragm.
- *Hiatal hernias* can weaken the barrier between the stomach and esophagus, facilitating the reflux of stomach acid and contributing to the development of heartburn.

## Dietary Habits:

- Individuals with obesity may be more prone to consuming larger meals, eating late at night, or consuming high-fat and acidic foods—common triggers for acid reflux.
- Unhealthy dietary habits associated with obesity can further contribute to the occurrence and severity of heartburn.

## Inflammatory Factors:

- Obesity is often accompanied by low-grade inflammation throughout the body, including the digestive system. Inflammation can affect the esophageal lining, making it more susceptible to irritation and damage from stomach acid.

Addressing obesity through lifestyle modifications, including weight loss, adopting a healthy diet, engaging in regular physical activity, and seeking medical guidance for weight management, can play a crucial role in managing and preventing heartburn.

These interventions aim to reduce the risk factors associated with obesity and promote overall digestive health.

# Smoking and Nicotine Use

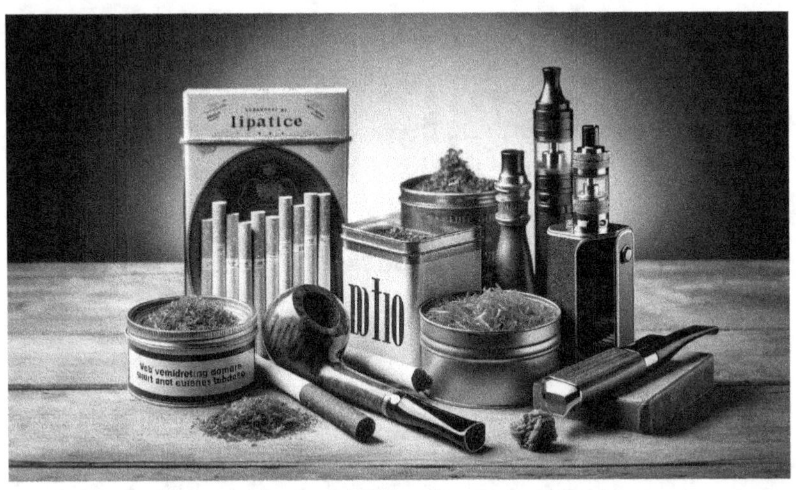

## <u>Nicotine can contribute to heartburn in several ways</u>
### (including Cigarettes, Cigars, Chew, Pipe Smoke, Vaping)

Firstly, nicotine relaxes the *lower esophageal sphincter* *(LES)*. When the *LES* is relaxed, it loses its ability to effectively prevent stomach acid from flowing back into the esophagus. This relaxation of the *LES* is a key factor in the development of acid reflux and subsequent heartburn.

## Relaxation of the Lower Esophageal Sphincter (LES):

- When the *LES* is relaxed, it becomes less effective in preventing stomach acid from flowing back into the *esophagus*.

## Increased Stomach Acid Production:
- Smoking stimulates the production of stomach acid.
- Elevated levels of stomach acid increase the likelihood of acid reflux, as the excess acid may flow back into the *esophagus*.

## Impaired Esophageal Function:
- Smoking can impair the normal function of the *esophagus*, making it more vulnerable to the damaging effects of stomach acid.
- The combination of nicotine's relaxing effect on the *LES* and increased stomach acid production creates an environment conducive to the development of heartburn.

## Reduced Salivation:
- Smoking can reduce saliva production.
- Saliva plays a role in neutralizing stomach acid. Reduced saliva levels can result in decreased acid neutralization, contributing to the irritation of the esophagus and heartburn.

## Inflammatory Response:

- Smoking is associated with inflammation throughout the body, including the digestive system.
- Inflammation in the *esophagus* can further exacerbate the symptoms of heartburn.

## An Encouraging Word...

Quitting smoking might seem like an impossible task, almost like trying to move a mountain with your bare hands. Nicotine's grip is tight, creating an addiction that's both physical and absolutely mental as well. It's not just about the chemical hooks; smoking becomes a part of who you are, a way to deal with stress, boredom, or social situations.

Smoking is intertwined with so many daily routines and activities, it's literally like trying to break 200 habits, not just one. After Meals, with coffee or alcohol, during breaks at work, while driving, socializing, when stressed, upon waking, during leisure activities etc. etc.

The key lies in understanding that quitting is a journey, not a single event. It's about arming yourself with the right tools— could be: nicotine replacement therapies, counseling, support from friends and family, but perhaps most importantly, a solid plan.

Every attempt to quit, even if it doesn't lead to immediate success, strengthens your resolve and brings you closer to your goal. Remember, the only way to truly fail is to stop trying. With each step forward, you're rewriting your story, proving that even the most daunting challenges can be overcome.

## <u>Cigarettes, Cigars, Chew, Pipe Smoke, Vaping</u>

**Making the decision to stop using tobacco in these many forms is a life-changing decision that brings about numerous health, financial, and social benefits.**

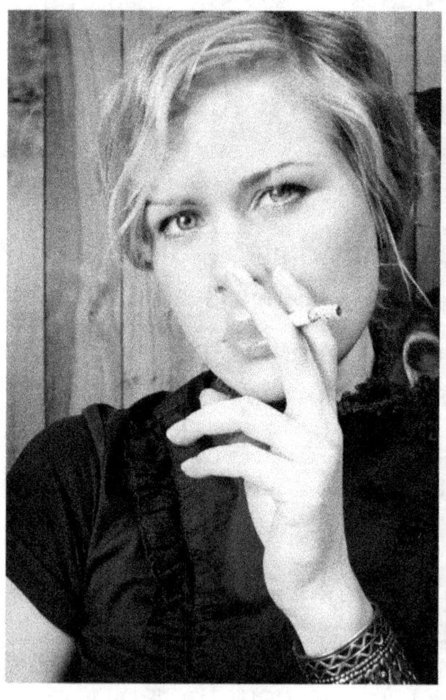 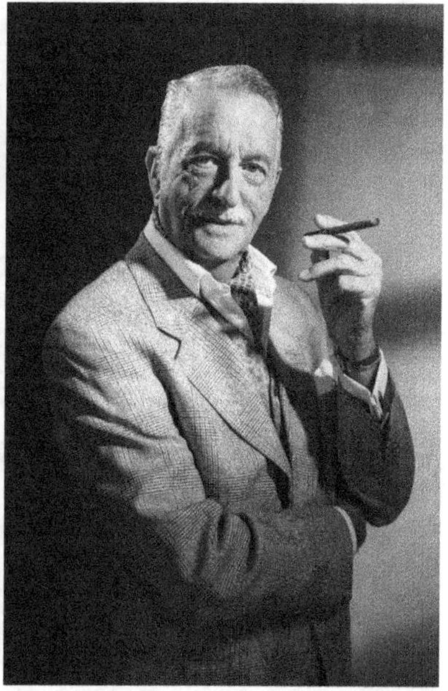

# <u>25 Additional Reasons to</u>
## <u>Stop Using Nicotine</u>

**1. Improved Respiratory Health:**
- Elimination of chronic coughing, wheezing, and shortness of breath.
- Reduced risk of respiratory conditions such as chronic bronchitis and emphysema.
- Enhanced lung function and capacity for physical activities.

**2. Reduced Risk of Cancer:**
- Lowered risk of developing various cancers, including lung, throat, mouth, esophagus, and bladder cancer.
- Improved chances of preventing cancer-related mortality.

**3. Enhanced Cardiovascular Health:**
- Reduced risk of heart disease, heart attacks, and strokes.
- Improved blood circulation and lowered blood pressure.

**4. Better Oral Health:**
- Decreased risk of gum disease, tooth decay, and tooth loss.
- Fresher breath and improved overall oral hygiene.

**5. Increased Energy Levels:**
- Improved stamina and endurance for physical activities.

- Better overall energy levels and reduced fatigue.

## 6. Enhanced Physical Fitness:
- Improved lung function leading to better athletic performance.
- Increased ability to engage in exercise and fitness routines.

## 7. Financial Savings:
- Significant cost savings by eliminating expenses on cigarettes.
- Opportunity to redirect money towards more meaningful and rewarding pursuits.

## 8. Improved Mental Health:
- Reduced levels of stress, anxiety, and depression.
- Better overall mental well-being and mood.

## 9. Enhanced Sense of Taste and Smell:
- Gradual restoration of taste and smell senses.
- Increased enjoyment of food and beverages..

## 10. Reduced Risk to Others (Secondhand Smoke):
- Protection of nonsmokers, especially children and pregnant women, from the harmful effects of secondhand smoke.
- Positive impact on the health of family members and those in close proximity.

## 11. Improved Skin Health:
- Slowed aging of the skin and reduction in wrinkles.
- Enhanced skin complexion and overall appearance.

## 12. Enhanced Fertility:
- Improved reproductive health in both men and women.
- Increased chances of successful conception.

## 13. Increased Life Expectancy:
- Numerous health benefits contributing to a longer life expectancy.
- Improved overall quality of life in the long term.

## 14. Positive Role Modeling:
- Serving as a positive example for family, friends, and the community.
- Inspiring others to make positive lifestyle changes.

## 15. Sense of Accomplishment:
- Overcoming the addiction to tobacco provides a sense of accomplishment.
- Boosted self-esteem and increased confidence.

## 16. Improved Social Life:
- Elimination of social stigma associated with smoking.
- Increased acceptance and inclusion in social activities.

17. **Better Sleep Quality:**
   - Reduced disruption to sleep patterns caused by nicotine.
   - Improved overall sleep quality and restfulness.

18. **Decreased Risk of Digestive Issues:**
   - Lowered risk of developing conditions like acid reflux and **Peptic Ulcers**.
   - Improved digestive health and comfort.

19. **Positive Impact on Chronic Conditions:**
   - Improved management of chronic conditions such as diabetes and hypertension.
   - Decreased severity of symptoms and complications.

20. **Healthier Aging Process:**
   - Slowed aging process and increased vitality.
   - Improved chances of aging with better health.

21. **Increased Immune System Function:**
   - Strengthened immune system, leading to better resistance to illnesses.
   - Reduced susceptibility to infections.

22. **Enhanced Smell and Breath:**
   - Elimination of tobacco odor from breath and clothing.
   - Fresher smelling breath and improved personal hygiene.

**23. Reduced Environmental Impact:**
- Decreased contribution to environmental pollution from cigarette butts.
- Positive impact on the environment and public spaces.

**24. Improved Cognitive Function:**
- Better cognitive abilities and mental sharpness.
- Reduced risk of cognitive decline and dementia.

**25. Freedom from Addiction:**
- Break from the cycle of addiction and dependence on nicotine.
- Freedom to live a life not dictated by the need for tobacco.

The path to quitting tobacco often involves a combination of several different strategies and persistent efforts. Here are a few hints and actions that may help you with this difficult yet achievable task:

☐ ***Personal Motivation:***

Key Factor: Internal motivation is crucial. A strong desire to quit, driven by health concerns, financial considerations, or personal goals, provides a foundation for success.

- [ ] ***Setting a Quit Date:***
Key Factor: Choosing a specific quit date creates a tangible goal and allows for mental preparation.

- [ ] ***Nicotine Replacement Therapy (NRT):***
Key Factor: Using NRT, such as patches, gum, or lozenges, helps manage withdrawal symptoms by providing controlled doses of nicotine.

- [ ] ***Behavioral Support:***
Key Factor: Seeking counseling, support groups, or behavioral therapy addresses the psychological aspects of addiction, providing coping mechanisms and encouragement.

- [ ] ***Prescription Medications:***
Key Factor: Medications like bupropion (Zyban) or varenicline (Chantix) prescribed by healthcare professionals can aid in reducing cravings and withdrawal symptoms.

- [ ] ***Avoiding Triggers:***
Key Factor: Identifying and avoiding situations or environments that trigger the desire to smoke helps break the habit loop (the 100 habits mentioned earlier).

- [ ] ***Healthy Lifestyle Changes:***
Key Factor: Adopting healthier habits, including regular exercise, balanced nutrition, and stress management, supports the overall quitting process.

☐ ***Support from Family and Friends:***

Key Factor: Informing and involving friends and family in the quitting process provides a strong support system and encouragement.

☐ ***Mindfulness and Stress Reduction:***

Key Factor: Incorporating mindfulness techniques, such as meditation or deep breathing, helps manage stress without resorting to tobacco use.

☐ ***Celebrate Milestones:***

Key Factor: Celebrating small victories and milestones reinforces the positive aspects of quitting and boosts motivation.

☐ ***Relapse Prevention Strategies:***

Key Factor: Developing strategies to handle potential setbacks or triggers is essential for preventing relapse.

☐ ***Professional Guidance:***

Key Factor: Seeking advice and support from healthcare professionals, including doctors, nurses, or quitlines, can provide personalized strategies and assistance.

Remember that the journey to quit nicotine use is unique for each individual. Success often comes from a combination of these factors, and persistence is key. If someone is struggling to quit, seeking professional help and adjusting strategies can enhance the likelihood of long-term success.

# Large Meals

Eating excessively large meals can contribute to heartburn. When you consume a large amount of food in one sitting, it can lead to increased pressure on *the lower esophageal sphincter (LES)*. The pressure on the *LES* may weaken its function, allowing stomach acid to flow back into the *esophagus*, causing heartburn.

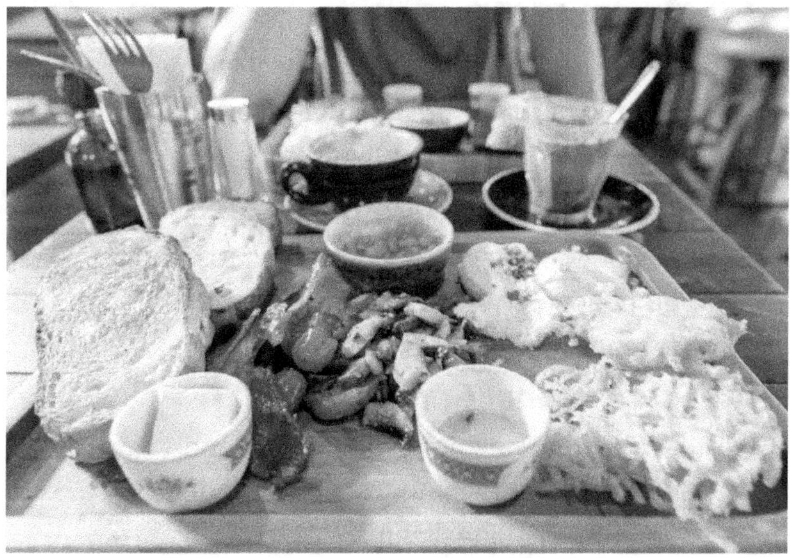

Additionally, large meals can lead to *delayed stomach emptying*, which means that the stomach takes longer to digest the food. This extended digestion process can increase the likelihood of stomach acid refluxing into the *esophagus* and causing discomfort.

To minimize the risk of heartburn, it's advisable to eat smaller, more frequent meals, choose foods that are less likely to trigger heartburn, and avoid lying down immediately after eating. If heartburn persists or becomes a recurring issue, it's recommended to consult with a healthcare professional for further evaluation and guidance.

## Consuming Foods and Beverages that Trigger Heartburn

Among the various triggers for heartburn, the one we have the most control over and that can have the biggest effect on us is our choice of diet, including the foods and beverages we decide to eat and drink.

For this reason, in the next significant segment of this book, named "Strategies for Relief," we will start by exploring foods and beverages commonly known to initiate heartburn. You might find many of them quite predictable. That's OK, sometimes a repetitive reminder can further empower us to make good healthy choices.

Foods and beverages that are high in fat, for instance, can lead to heartburn by relaxing the *lower esophageal sphincter (LES)*. Similarly, spicy foods, citrus fruits, chocolate, full-fat dairy products,  mint, garlic, onions, and caffeinated or carbonated beverages can also cause the *LES* to relax, increasing the likelihood of acid reflux and heartburn.

As previously discussed, overeating or consuming large meals can put extra pressure on the stomach, forcing acid back up into the *esophagus*. Eating too quickly or lying down immediately after a meal can exacerbate these effects, leading to more frequent and severe episodes of heartburn.

Understanding the link between diet and heartburn is crucial for managing and preventing the discomfort it brings. By identifying and avoiding foods and beverages that trigger their symptoms, individuals can significantly reduce the frequency and intensity of heartburn episodes, improving their quality of life and overall digestive health.

# STRATEGIES FOR RELIEF

## FIVE
## Foods to Avoid

Let's look at some widely recognized food triggers for acid reflux and why you may want to consider avoiding them.

## **Citrus Fruits**

While rich in vitamin C and other nutrients, citrus fruits are naturally acidic, containing citric acid. This acidity can contribute to a lower pH in the stomach, potentially leading to irritation of the *esophagus* and the development or worsening of heartburn symptoms.

In addition, the *LES* may relax, allowing stomach acid to flow back into the *esophagus* and causing heartburn.

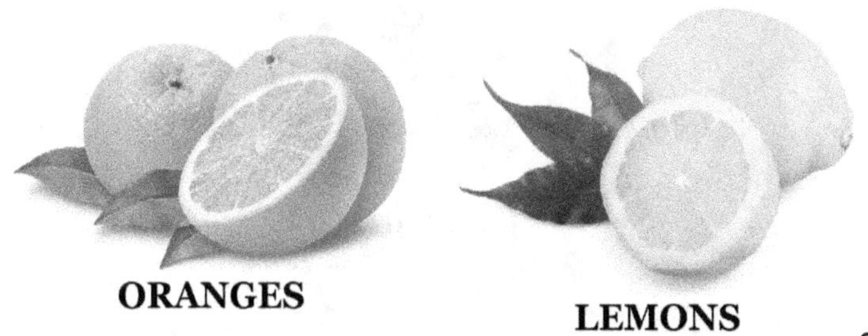

Consumption of acidic foods, including citrus fruits, can stimulate the stomach to produce more acid. Excessive stomach acid increases the likelihood of acid reflux into the esophagus.

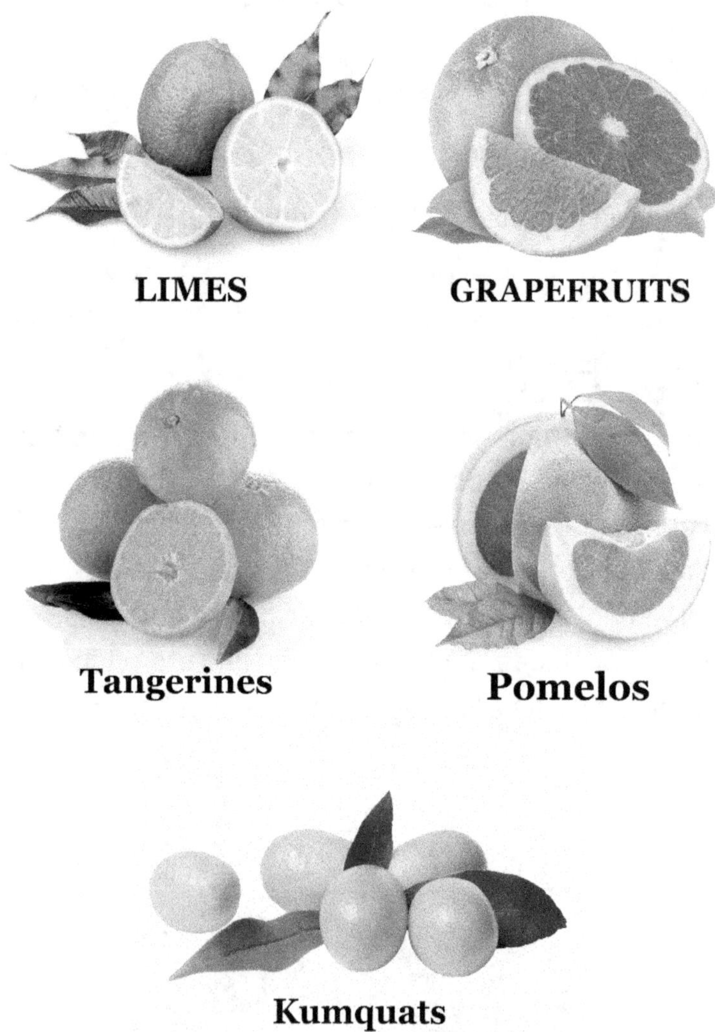

# Tomatoes and Tomato Products

Tomato products can cause heartburn due to their high acidity. Tomatoes contain citric and *Malic Acids*, which can trigger the release of stomach acid and relax the *lower esophageal sphincter (LES)*. This relaxation allows stomach acid to flow back into the *esophagus*, causing irritation and the characteristic burning sensation of heartburn.

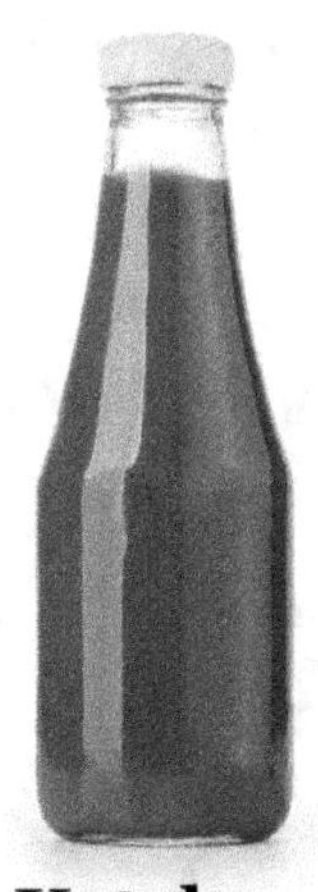

**Ketchup**

Additionally, tomatoes contain a compound called *Lycopene*, which may contribute to acid reflux in some individuals. Cooking processes, like canning, may also concentrate acidity in tomato products, making them more likely to cause heartburn.

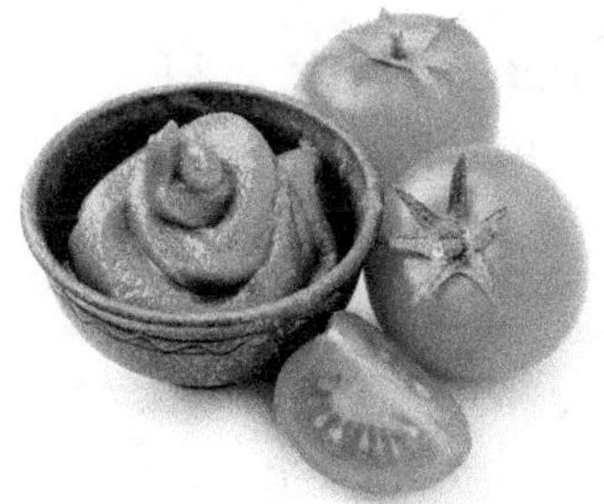

**Tomatoes**

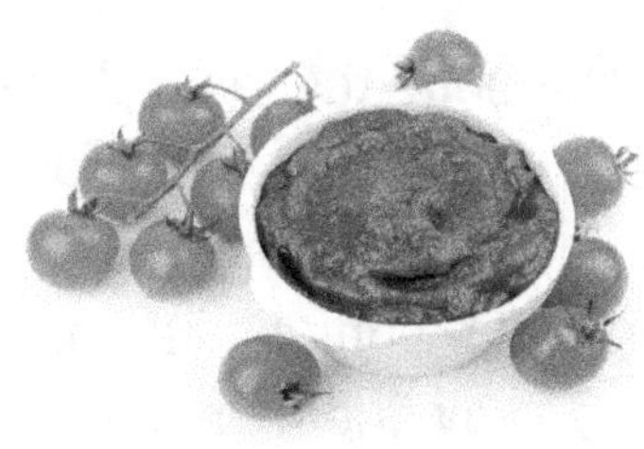

**Paste**

# Onions and Garlic

Onions and garlic contain compounds that can contribute to heartburn. Both are rich in sulfur-containing compounds and fructans, which can irritate the *esophagus* and lead to *(LES)* relaxation. This relaxation allows stomach acid to flow back into the *esophagus*, causing the characteristic burning sensation of heartburn.

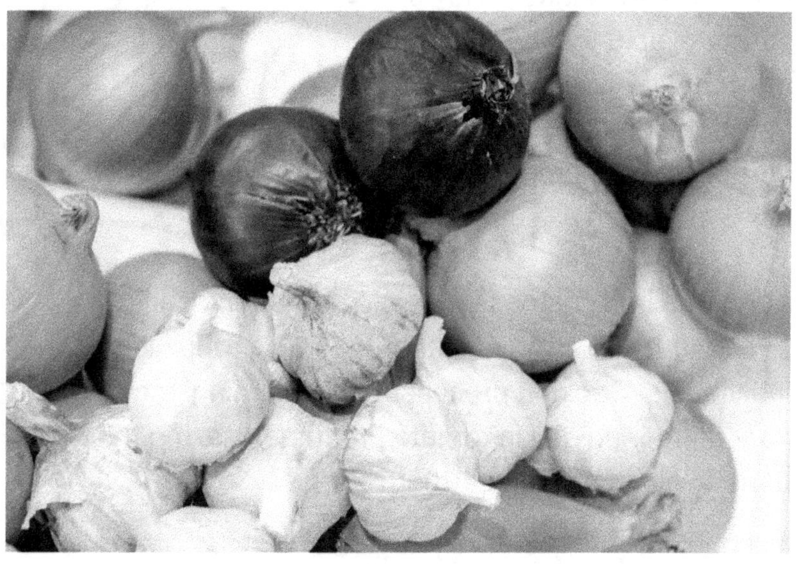

Additionally, these foods can increase gastric acid production, further exacerbating the risk of acid reflux. While not everyone may experience heartburn after consuming onions and garlic, individuals prone to acid reflux may find it beneficial to moderate their intake of these flavorful but potentially triggering ingredients.

# Full Fat Dairy

Full-fat dairy products can contribute to heartburn due to their high fat content. High-fat foods can also significantly relax the (*LES*).

When the *LES* is relaxed, stomach acid can flow back into the *esophagus*, leading to discomfort. Additionally, fatty foods delay stomach emptying, allowing acid to remain in the stomach for a more extended period, increasing the likelihood of reflux.

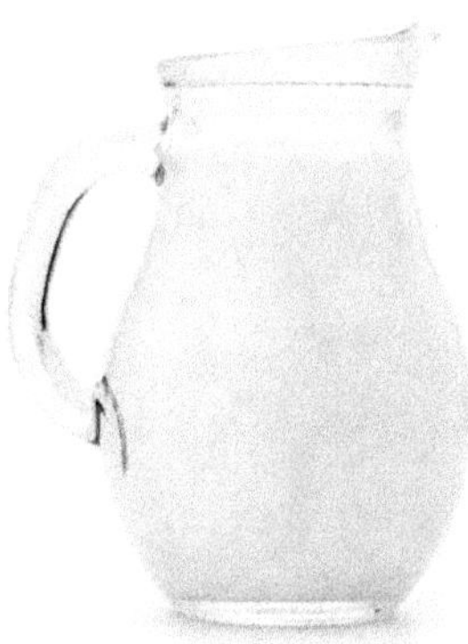

**Whole Milk**

While not everyone experiences heartburn from full-fat dairy, individuals prone to acid reflux may find relief by opting for lower-fat dairy alternatives to reduce the risk of symptoms.

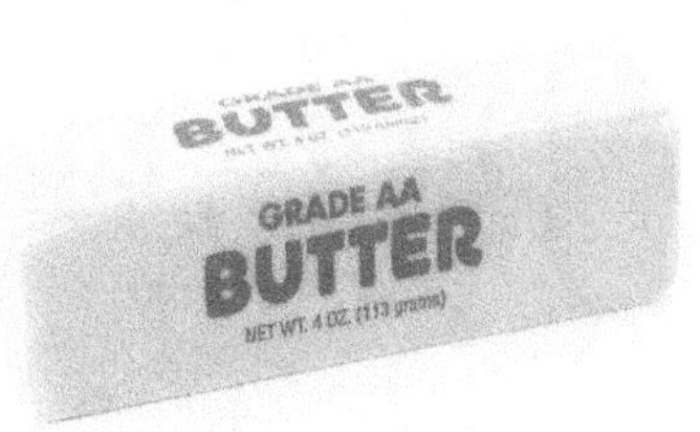


**Non Reduced-Fat Butter**

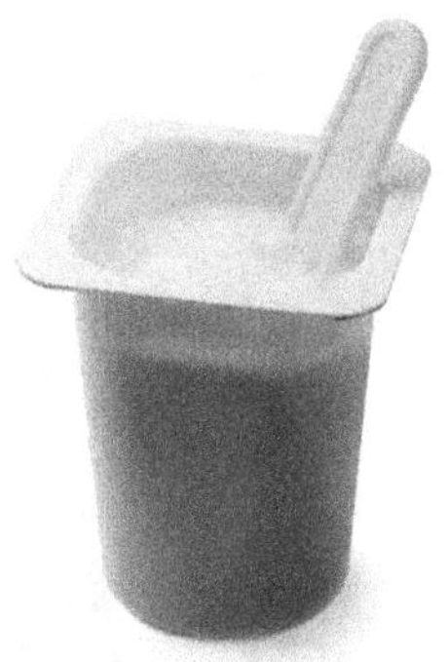

**Full Fat Yogurt**

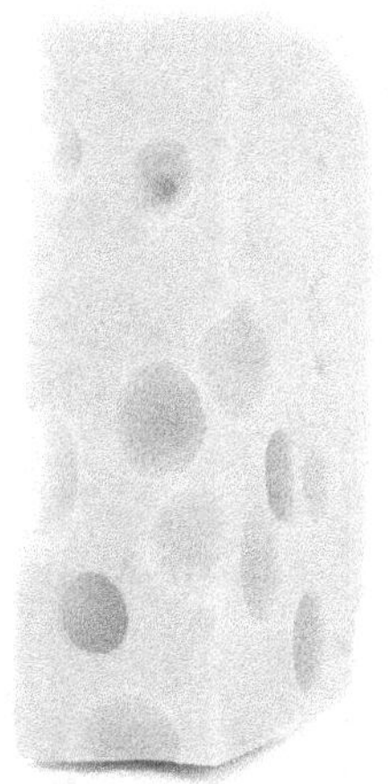

**Varieties of Cheese**

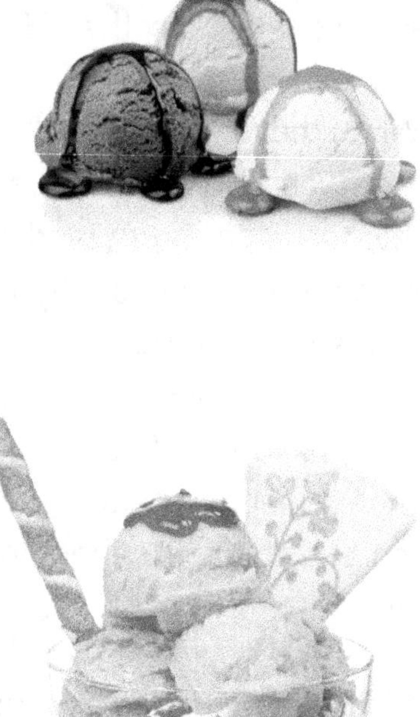

**Ice Cream**

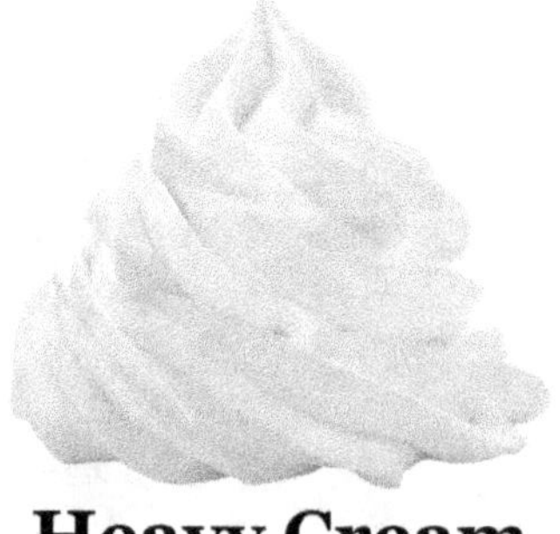

**Heavy Cream**

# Fatty Meats

Fatty meats can contribute to heartburn due to their high fat content. High-fat foods, including fatty meats, relax (*LES*). When the *LES* is weakened, similar to high fat dairy products and citrus foods. Stomach acid can reflux into the *esophagus*.

Additionally, fatty foods tend to slow down the emptying of the stomach, prolonging the time stomach acid is in contact with the *esophagus*. Individuals prone to acid reflux may experience relief by choosing leaner meat options to minimize the risk of heartburn.

**Examples of fatty meats include cuts that contain higher amounts of visible fat or marbling within the meat. Some examples are:**

> **Fatty Cuts of Beef:**
> - Ribeye steak
> - T-bone steak
> - New York strip steak
>
> **Fatty Cuts of Pork:**
> - Pork belly
> - Spareribs
> - Bacon
>
> **Processed Meats:**
> - Sausages
> - Hot dogs
> - Bologna

**Dark Poultry Meat:**
- Chicken thighs with skin
- Duck
- Goose

It's important to note that while these meats may be higher in fat, not all fats are unhealthy. Some cuts of meat, particularly those containing *monounsaturated* and *polyunsaturated fats*, can be part of a balanced diet. However, moderation and choosing leaner options are often recommended for overall health, especially for individuals looking to manage their fat intake.

# A Few Samples of "fatty" Meats

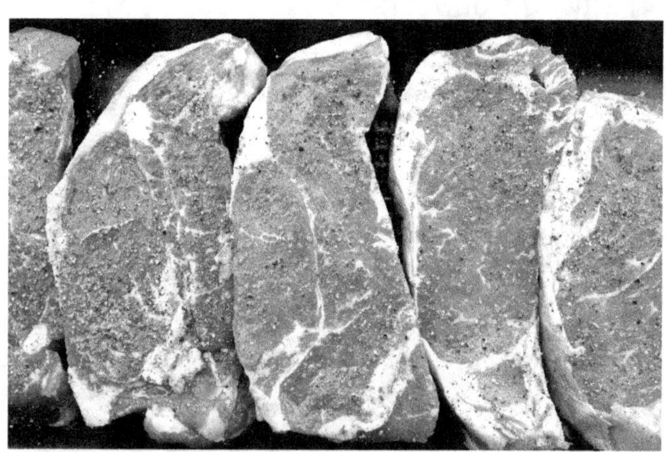

# New York Steaks

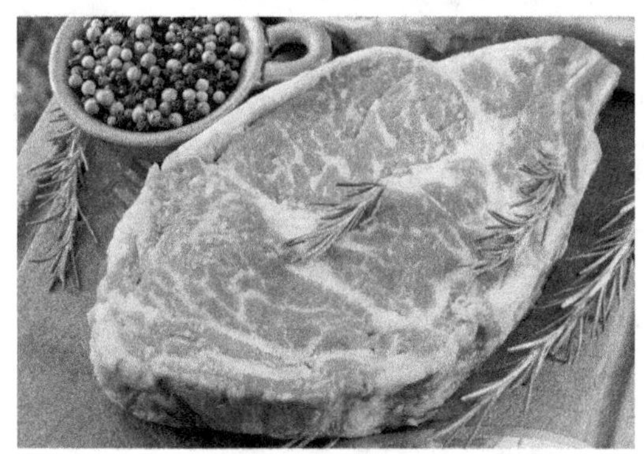

**Ribe-Eye**

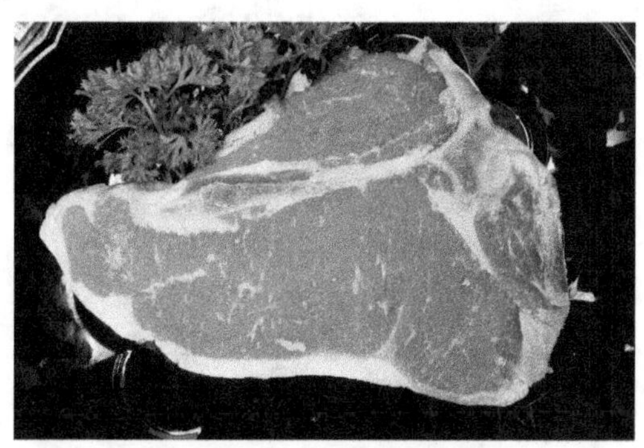

**T-Bone Steak**

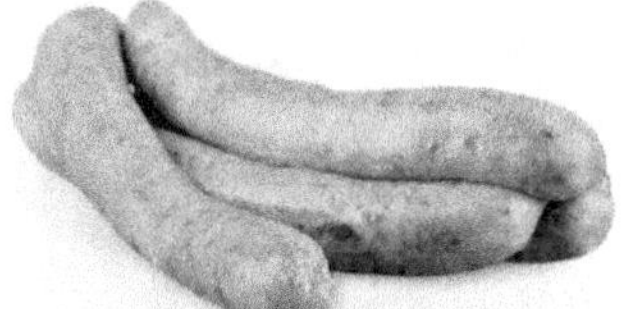

**Sausage**

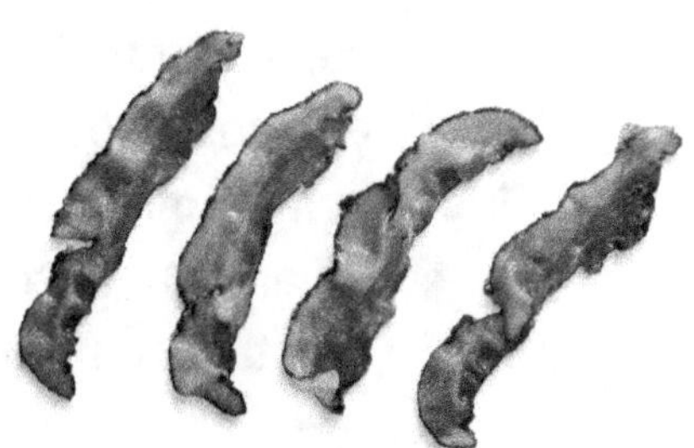

**Bacon**

# Fatty and Fried Foods

Fatty and fried foods include items that are high in unhealthy fats and are often deep-fried or cooked in oil. These foods, though delicious, are typically associated with higher calorie and fat content. Some examples are:

**French Fries:**
- Potatoes cut into strips and deep-fried until crispy.

**Fried Chicken:**
- Chicken pieces coated in batter or breadcrumbs and deep-fried.

**Onion Rings:**
- Sliced onions coated in batter and deep-fried until golden brown.

**Fried Mozzarella Sticks:**
- Breaded and fried sticks of mozzarella cheese.

**Doughnuts:**
- Sweet fried dough pastries are often coated in sugar or glaze.

**Chips and Nachos:**
- Potato chips or tortilla chips are often served with high-fat toppings like cheese and sour cream.

**Fried Spring Rolls or Egg Rolls:**
- Asian appetizers filled with vegetables, meat, or seafood and deep-fried.

**Fried Calamari:**
- Squid rings coated in batter and deep-fried.

**Fried Pastries:**
- Various pastries, such as fried pies or fritters, filled with sweet or savory ingredients.

**Fried Fish and Seafood:**
- Fish or seafood coated in batter or breadcrumbs and deep-fried.

While these foods can be enjoyed in moderation, a diet high in fried and fatty foods may contribute to health issues such as weight gain and increased risk of heart disease.

It's advisable to balance such indulgences with a diet rich in fruits, vegetables, lean proteins, and whole grains for overall health and well-being.

# A Few Samples of "fatty & Fried" Foods

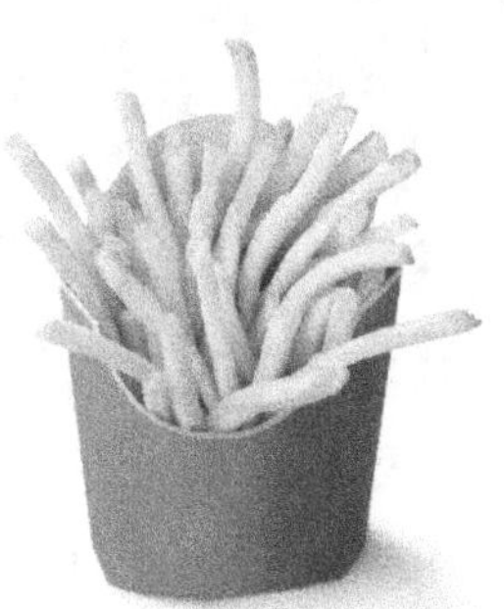

**French Fries**

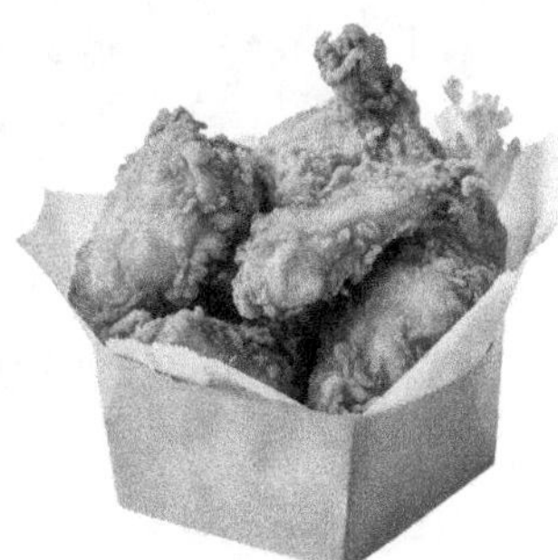

**Fried Chicken**

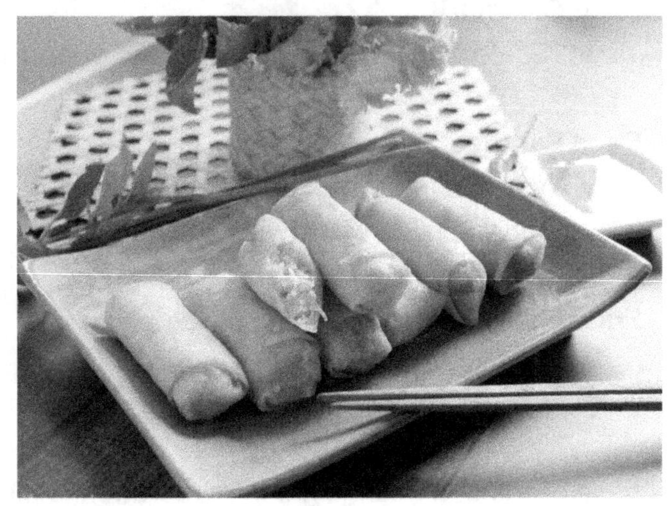

**Fried Spring Rolls or Egg Rolls**

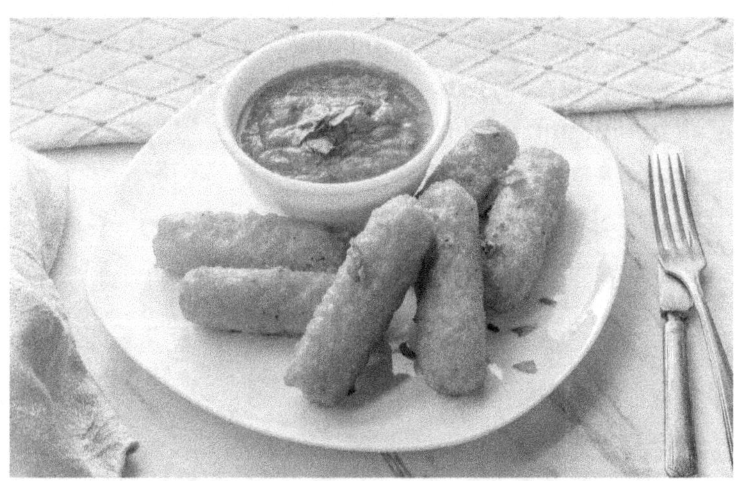

**Fried Mozzarella Sticks**

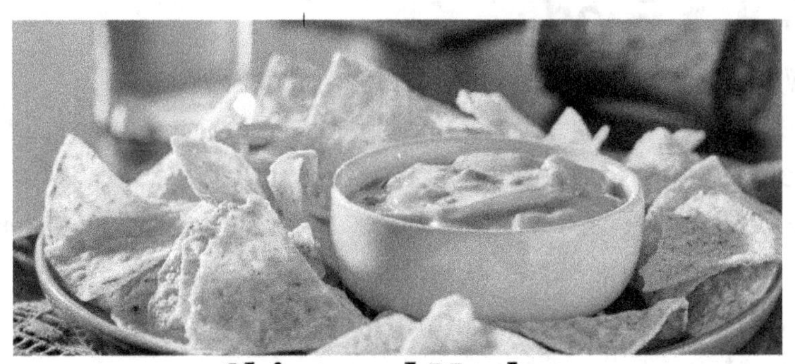

# Chips and Nachos

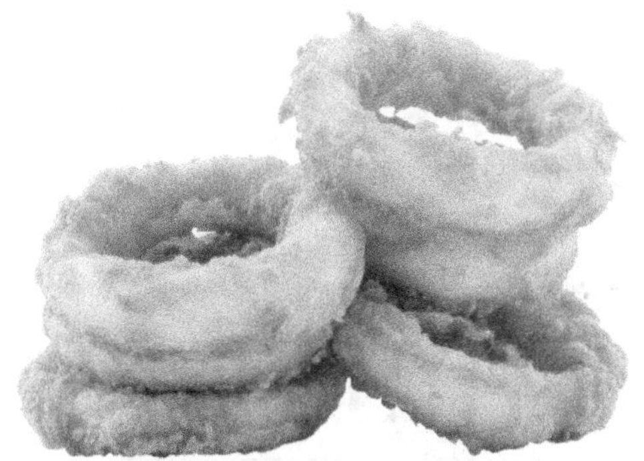

# Onion Rings

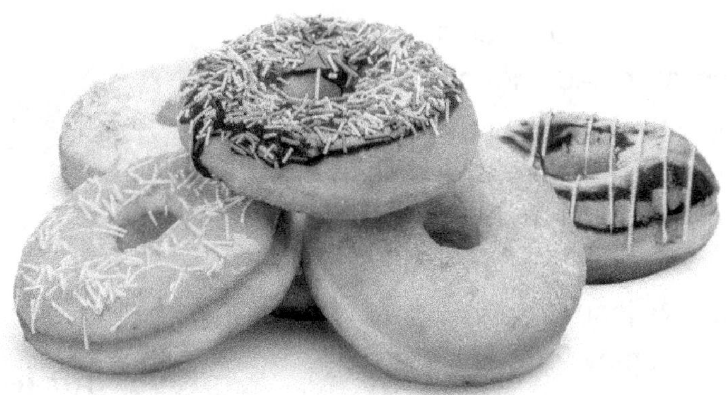

# Doughnuts

# Spicy Foods

While spicy foods can add flavor, they may not be suitable for everyone. Consuming excessive spicy foods, containing compounds like *Capsaicin*, can lead to digestive discomfort, heartburn, and irritation. Individuals with conditions like acid reflux, *Irritable Bowel Syndrome (IBS)*, or gastritis may experience worsened symptoms.

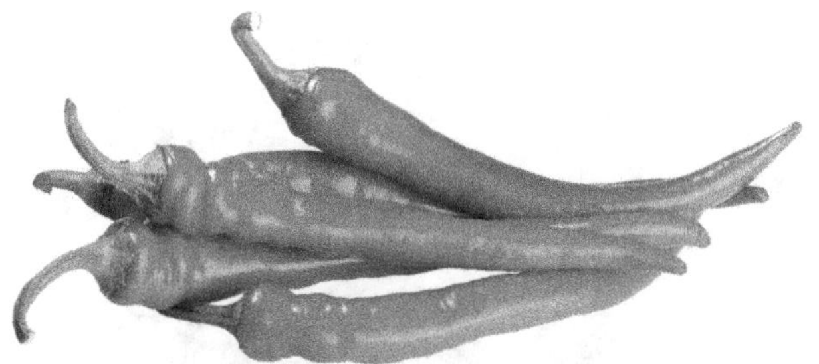

**Chili Peppers**

Spicy foods can also contribute to sleep disturbances and discomfort. Additionally, some people may have a lower tolerance to heat, making spicy foods unpleasant. Moderation is key, and those with pre-existing digestive issues should consider limiting spicy food intake to maintain digestive comfort and overall well-being.

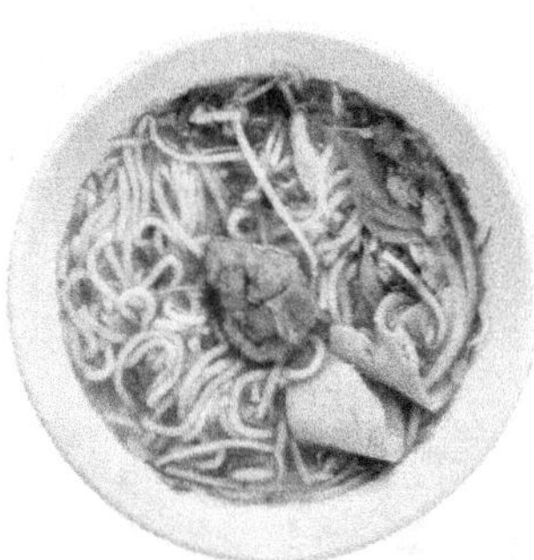

**Spicy Noodles**

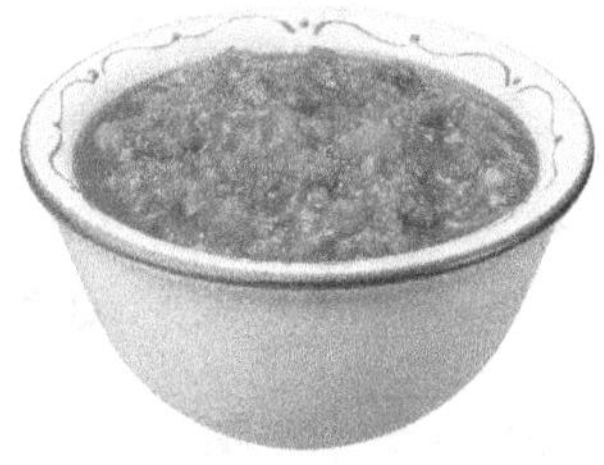

Salsa

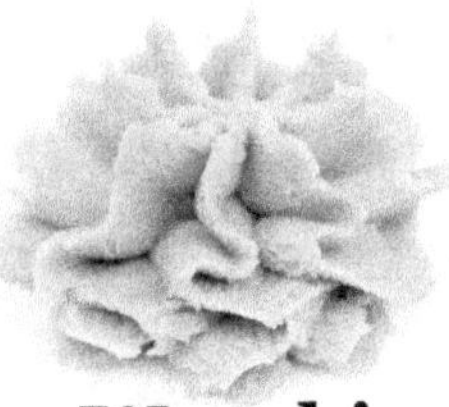

Wasabi

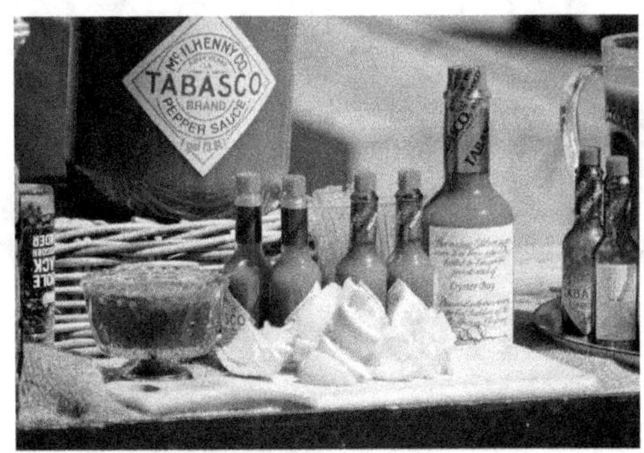

## Hot Sauces

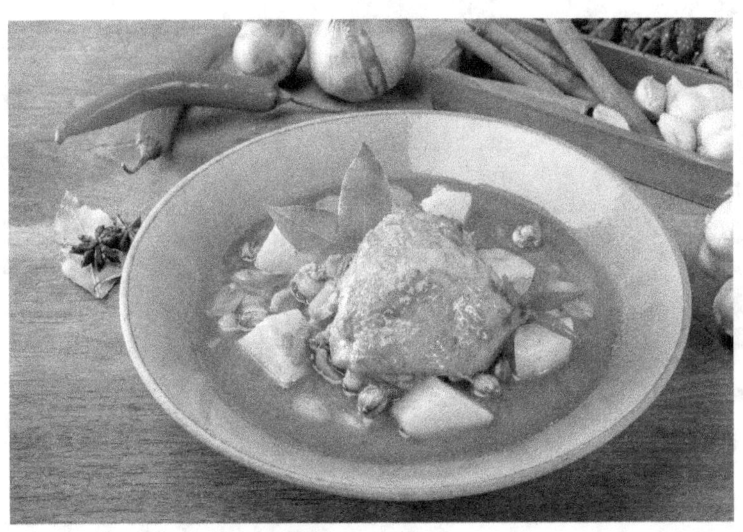

## Curries

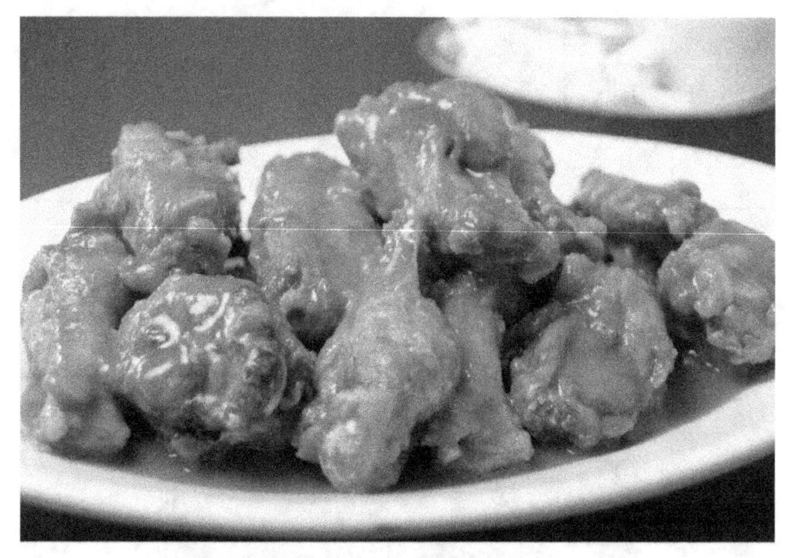

# Buffalo Wings

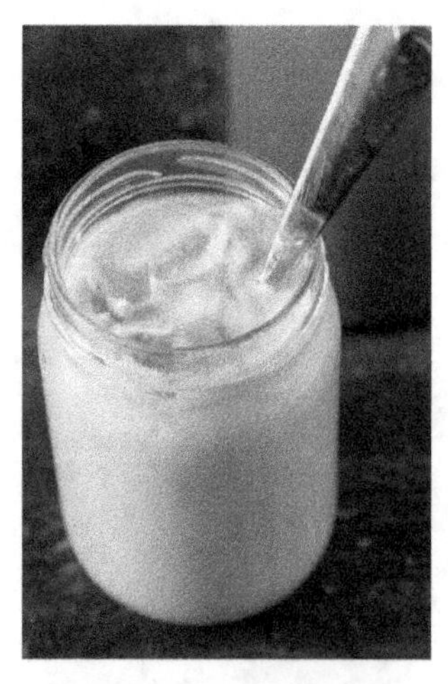

**Hot Mustard**

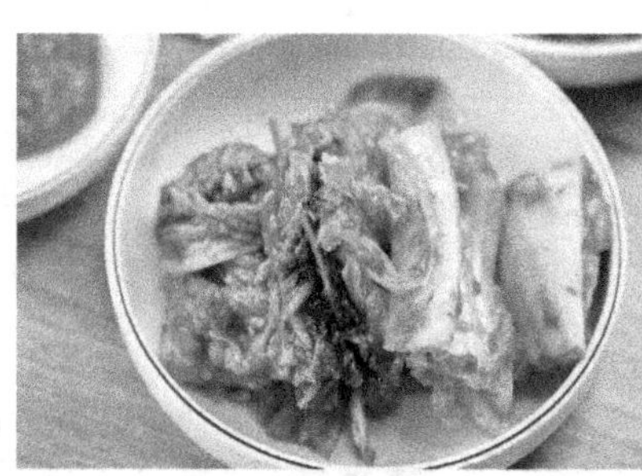

**Kimchi**

# Processed Foods

Processed foods are food items that have undergone various alterations from their original state through methods such as cooking, canning, freezing, or packaging. These alterations are intended to enhance the taste, texture, shelf life, or convenience of the food product.

However, they are often detrimental to health due to their high levels of added sugars, unhealthy fats, and sodium. These components contribute to conditions such as obesity, hypertension, and heart disease, and of course heartburn. The processing itself can lead to the removal of essential nutrients, diminishing the nutritional value of the food.

The spectrum of processed foods ranges from minimally processed items to highly refined and heavily processed products, each with its own set of implications for nutrition and health.

**Minimally processed foods** are those that have undergone the least amount of modification. Examples include washed and pre-cut fruits and vegetables, bagged salads, and roasted nuts. These foods typically retain much of their original nutritional content.

**Moderately processed foods** undergo more substantial changes but still maintain some of their original nutritional value. This category includes foods like canned vegetables, whole grain bread, and freshly squeezed fruit juices.

**Highly processed foods** undergo significant modifications and often involve the addition of various ingredients for flavor enhancement, preservation, or texture improvement. Examples include ready-to-eat meals, sugary snacks, sodas, and certain convenience foods.

## Key Characteristics of Processed Foods:

➤ **Additives:** Many processed foods contain additives such as preservatives, sweeteners, colorings, and flavor enhancers. These substances aim to improve the product's appearance, taste, and shelf life.
However, they can be unhealthy for various reasons. Some additives, like artificial sweeteners and colors, have been associated with adverse reactions such as headaches and allergies.

Certain preservatives, like *BHA* and *BHT*, have raised concerns about potential long-term health risks. High levels of sodium in additives like *Monosodium Glutamate (MSG)* may contribute to *Hypertension*. Additionally, the cumulative effect of various additives in processed foods may pose health concerns when consumed in excess.

➤ **Refinement:** Processing often involves refining grains, removing the bran and germ. While this enhances shelf life, it also eliminates essential nutrients like fiber, vitamins, and minerals.

➤ **Convenience:** Processed foods are designed for convenience, offering quick and easy meal solutions. This aspect of convenience can be appealing to individuals with busy lifestyles.

➤ **Packaging:** Processed foods are commonly found in various forms of packaging, from cans and boxes to plastic containers. Packaging serves not only as a means of preservation but also for marketing and consumer appeal.

➤ **High Levels of Salt, Sugar, and Unhealthy Fats:** High levels of salt, sugar, and unhealthy fats in processed foods contribute to a myriad of health issues. Excessive salt intake is linked to *hypertension* and increased risk of cardiovascular diseases. Consuming foods rich in added sugars is associated with weight gain, diabetes, and dental problems. Unhealthy fats, especially trans fats, raise bad cholesterol levels, contributing to heart disease. The combination of these components in processed foods not only undermines nutritional quality but also promotes unhealthy eating patterns, fostering a range of chronic conditions.

**Nutritional Implications:** Nutrient loss in processed foods is detrimental to health as it diminishes the nutritional value of the diet. Processing often involves refining grains, stripping away essential nutrients like fiber, vitamins, and minerals. This loss compromises the overall nutrient density of the food, potentially leading to nutrient deficiencies.

Adequate nutrient intake is crucial for maintaining optimal health, supporting bodily functions, and preventing various deficiencies and related health issues. Choosing whole, minimally processed foods ensures a more nutrient-rich and balanced approach to nutrition

➤ **Caloric Density:** Some processed foods are extremely energy-dense, meaning they provide a high number of calories without offering substantial nutritional value. They often lack essential nutrients like vitamins and minerals but are rich in unhealthy fats, sugars, and additives.

Consuming items with poor caloric density can contribute not only to weight gain, but oftentimes health issues due to the lack of delivering the necessary nutrients for overall well-being.

➤ **Added Sugars:** Processed foods, especially sweetened beverages, candies, and baked goods, often contain added sugars. Regular consumption of these items has been linked to an increased risk of metabolic issues and chronic diseases.

➤ **Sodium Intake:** Processed foods are often high in sodium, posing potential health risks. Excessive sodium intake is linked to *hypertension*, a major risk factor for heart disease and stroke. Many processed and packaged foods, such as canned soups, snacks, and ready-to-eat meals, contain elevated levels of salt for flavor enhancement and preservation.

Regularly consuming these items can contribute to an imbalance in sodium levels, leading to increased blood pressure. Monitoring and limiting sodium intake by choosing fresh, whole foods and checking food labels can help maintain a healthier diet and reduce the risk of cardiovascular issues associated with high sodium consumption.

## Balancing Processed Foods in the Diet:

While processed foods offer convenience, they can be detrimental when trying to reduce the incidents of heartburn/acid reflux. It's essential to strike a balance and prioritize a diet rich in whole, minimally processed foods. Here are some tips for making healthier choices:

### Read Labels:

- Check food labels for ingredients and nutritional information. Be mindful of added sugars, sodium content, and the presence of artificial additives.

**Choose Whole Foods:**

- Emphasize whole foods like fruits, vegetables, whole grains, lean proteins, and nuts. These provide essential nutrients and fiber without the additives found in many processed options.

**Limit Ultra-Processed Foods:**

- Reduce the consumption of highly processed and ultra-processed foods, as they tend to be high in unhealthy fats, sugars, and additives.

**Prepare Meals at Home:**

- Cooking meals at home allows for better control over ingredients and reduces reliance on heavily processed foods.

**Opt for Fresh or Frozen Produce:**

- Choose fresh or frozen fruits and vegetables over canned options. Fresh produce is less processed, and frozen varieties retain nutrients well.

**Moderation:**

- Enjoy processed foods in moderation. While it's okay to indulge occasionally, it's crucial to maintain a balanced diet overall.

# Conclusion:

Processed foods play a significant role in modern diets, offering convenience and accessibility. However, their nutritional impact varies, and some heavily processed options may contribute to health concerns when consumed excessively. Striking a balance by incorporating whole, minimally processed foods and being mindful of ingredient labels can help individuals make healthier choices and maintain a well-rounded diet. Ultimately, an emphasis on fresh, nutrient-dense foods forms the foundation of a balanced and nourishing eating pattern, thus reducing the frequency of heartburn.

## A Few Processed Foods

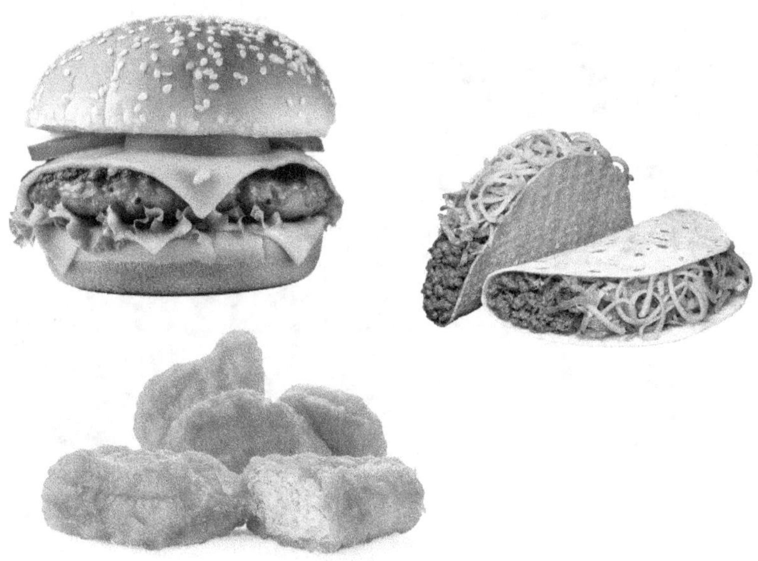

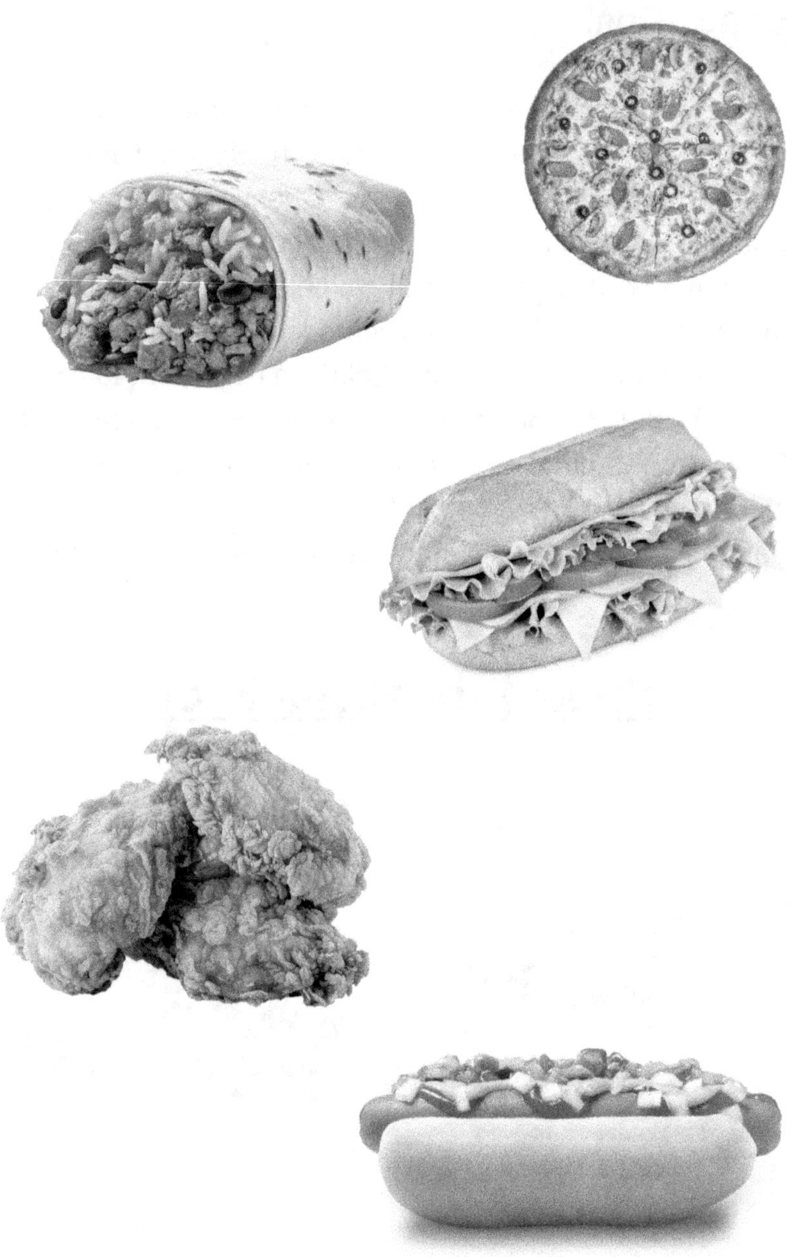

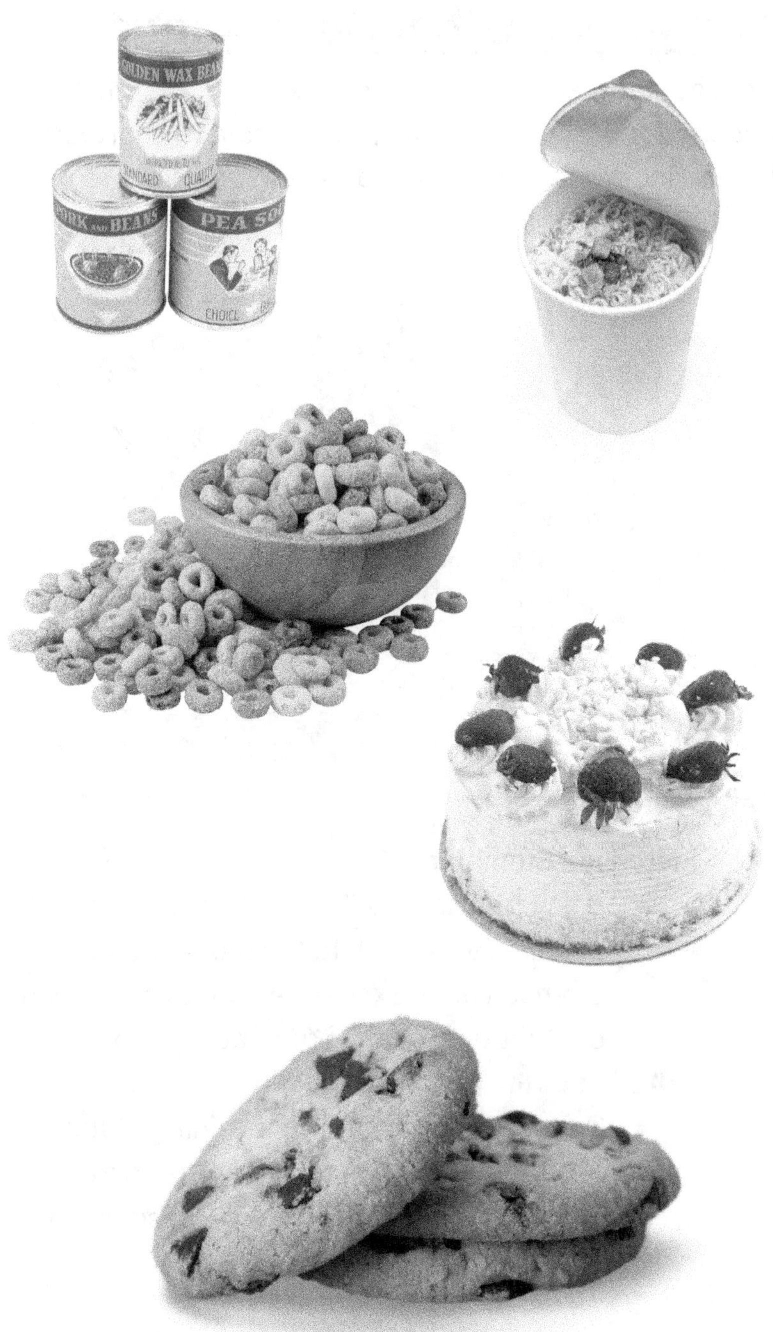

# Pepper and Other Seasonings

Pepper and other seasonings, including spicy or highly seasoned foods, can potentially contribute to heartburn in some individuals. Here are some reasons why:

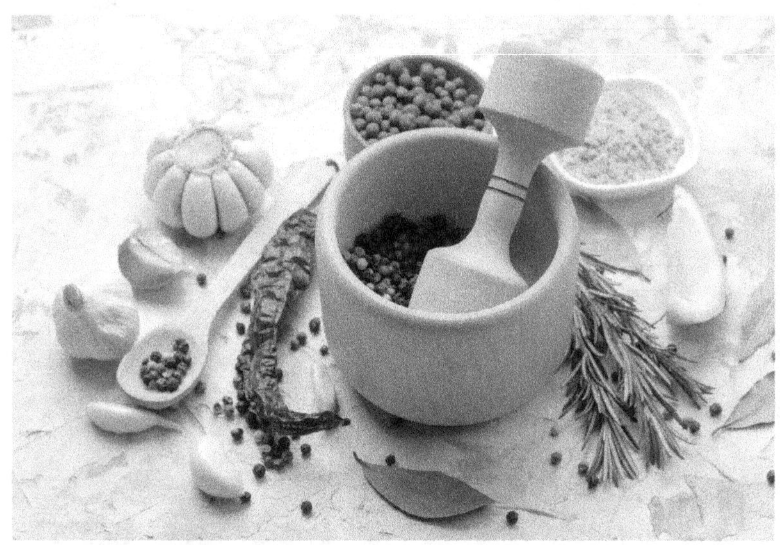

**Increased Stomach Acid:**
- Spicy foods, including those seasoned with pepper, can stimulate the production of stomach acid. Excessive stomach acid can contribute to heartburn or acid reflux.

**Irritation of the Esophagus:**
- Spicy foods may irritate the lining of the *esophagus*, leading to discomfort and a burning sensation, commonly associated with heartburn.

**Relaxation of the Lower Esophageal Sphincter (LES):**
- Some spicy foods may cause the *LES* to relax, allowing stomach acid to flow back into the esophagus.

**Individual Sensitivity:**
- Each person's tolerance to spices varies. While some individuals may experience heartburn after consuming spicy foods, others may not be affected.

By moderating seasoning intake, individuals can safeguard their digestive systems, allowing for a more comfortable and balanced culinary experience. Striking this balance not only promotes physical well-being but also enhances the enjoyment of diverse flavors in meals. It underscores the importance of mindful eating, encouraging individuals to savor their food while respecting the delicate equilibrium required for optimal digestive function.

# SIX

# Beverages to Avoid

## **Coffee and Caffeinated Beverages**

Coffee beverages, especially those containing caffeine, can cause heartburn due to their impact on the digestive system. Caffeine in coffee (as well as other caffeinated drinks) have a relaxing effect on the *(LES)*, causing stomach acid to flow back into the *esophagus*, causing heartburn.

Additionally, coffee stimulates the stomach to produce more acid, making the digestive environment more acidic. This increased acidity, combined with the relaxed *LES*, creates conditions favorable to the backward flow of stomach contents into the esophagus.

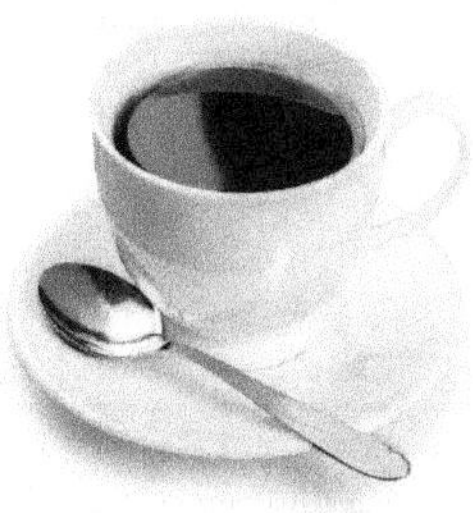

For individuals susceptible to heartburn, reducing coffee consumption, especially if it's high in caffeine, or opting for decaffeinated alternatives may help manage symptoms and promote digestive comfort.

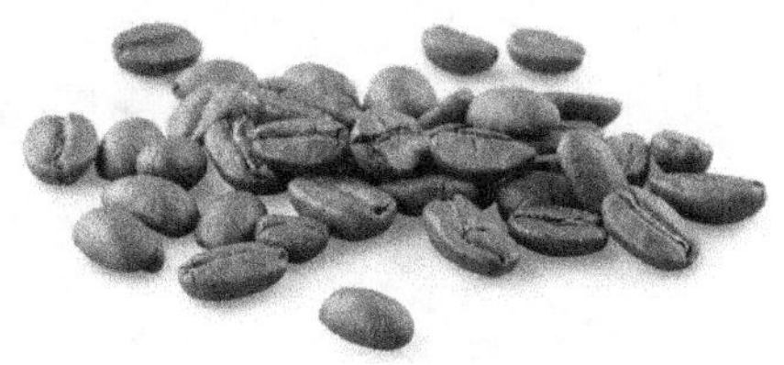

# Citrus Juices

Citrus juices, like orange, lemon or grapefruit juice, can contribute to heartburn due to their acidic nature. When consumed, the acidity of these juices can irritate the lining of the *esophagus*, leading to irritation and heartburn.

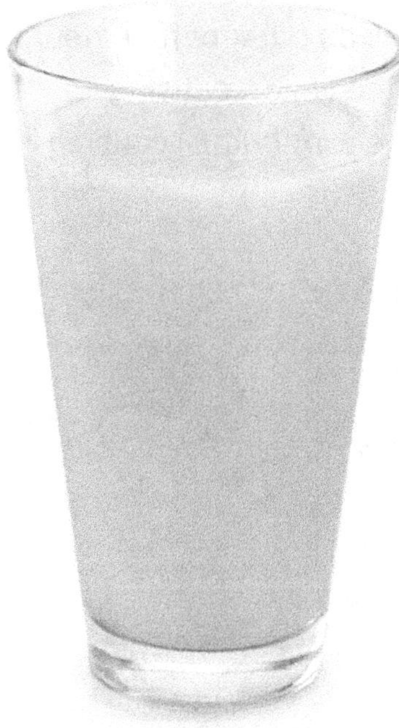

While citrus juices are rich in vitamins and flavors, individuals susceptible to heartburn may experience relief by moderating their intake or opting for less acidic alternatives. Understanding the impact of acidic foods on the digestive system can empower individuals to make dietary choices that promote comfort and well-being.

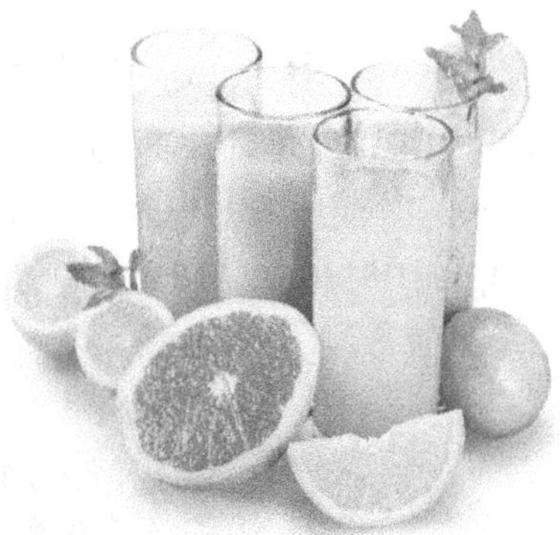

# Carbonated Drinks

Carbonated drinks, such as sodas, can contribute to heartburn due to their unique characteristics. The fizziness in these beverages is caused by carbon dioxide, which, when consumed, can create gas in the stomach. This gas can increase pressure in the stomach, leading to the relaxation of the *LES*.

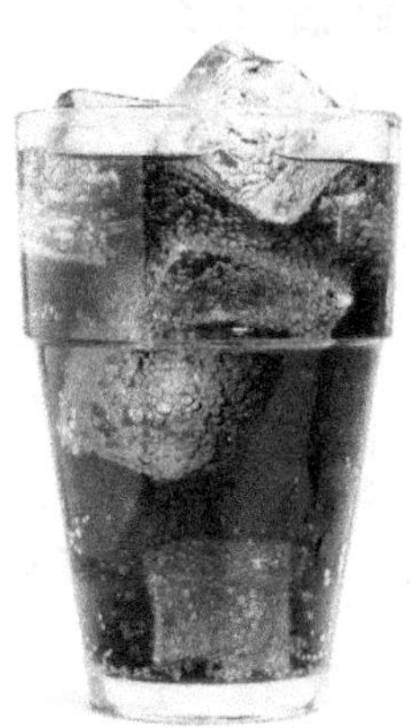

Additionally, the acidity of carbonated drinks can directly contribute to irritation in the *esophagus*. For individuals prone to heartburn, choosing non-carbonated alternatives or consuming carbonated beverages in moderation may help manage symptoms and promote digestive comfort.

Gaining insight into the impact of how carbonated beverages work on the digestive system helps us to make informed decisions about what we drink.

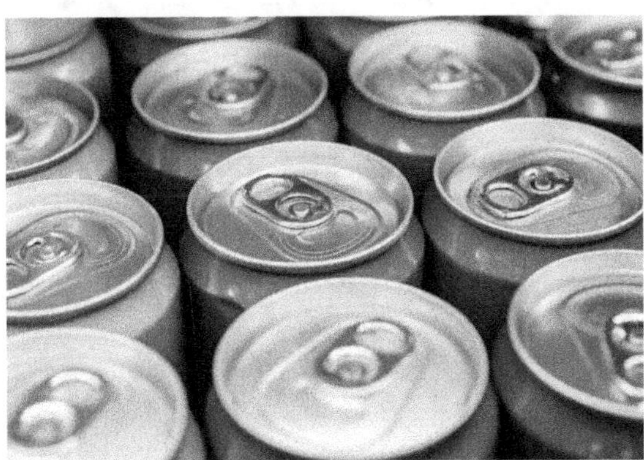

# Alcohol

For the purpose of this discussion, we'll focus solely on the physiological reasons alcohol causes heartburn, setting aside its broader implications.

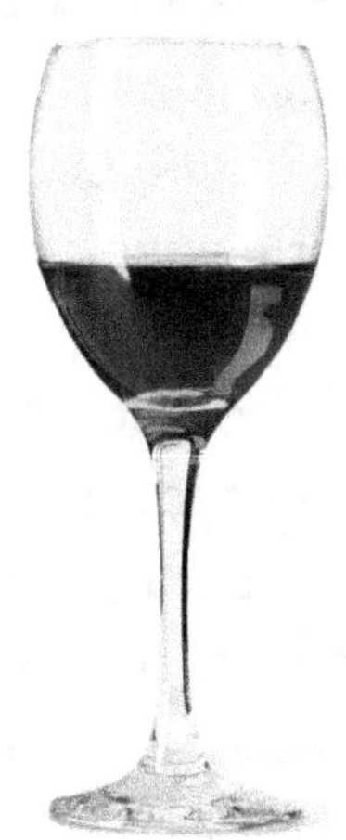

Drinking alcohol oftentimes can lead to heartburn due to its impact on the digestive system. Alcohol, like citrus drinks and coffee, also relaxes the *LES* which allows stomach acid to easily flow back into the throat passage.

Furthermore, alcohol will stimulate the stomach to produce more acid. The combination of a relaxed *esophagus* muscle and heightened acid production can create painful heartburn particularly on an empty stomach. Individuals more prone to acid reflux may experience relief by moderating alcohol intake, especially before bedtime, and being aware of their individual tolerance levels.

Being aware of these impacts enables individuals to make informed decisions about alcohol intake, promoting digestive comfort through conscious choices.

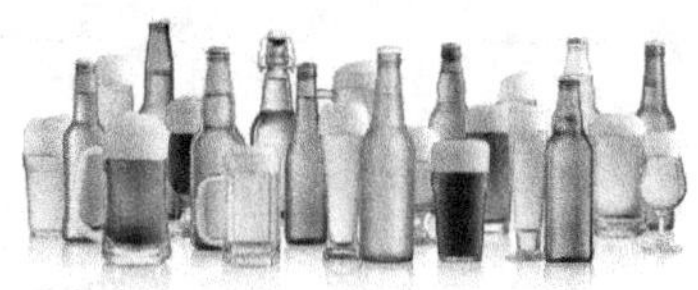

# Energy Drinks

Energy drinks can cause severe heartburn discomfort as well, with almost every factor often making up their content, caffeine, citric acid, sugars, carbonation and more.

Energy drinks are typically formulated with a combination of ingredients to provide a quick boost of energy and alertness. The primary components include caffeine, often derived from natural sources like coffee beans or synthetic sources, and sugar or artificial sweeteners for added sweetness. Additional ingredients may include amino acids, vitamins, and herbal extracts believed to enhance physical and mental performance.

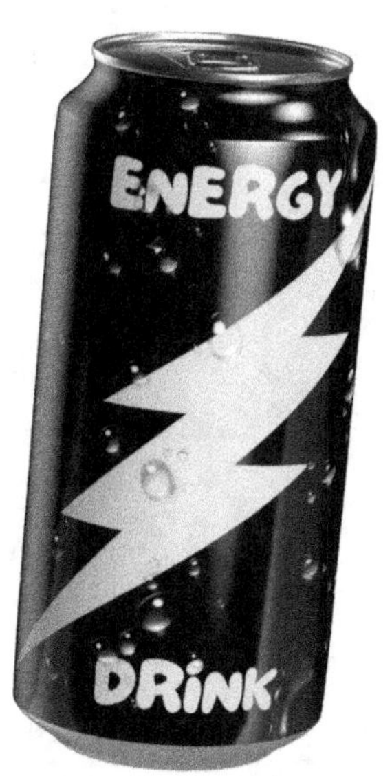


These ingredients are dissolved or mixed into a flavored liquid base, which oftentimes are carbonated. Preservatives and stabilizers are also usually added to extend shelf life. The final product is then packaged in cans or bottles. The formulation and production processes can vary among brands, each aiming to create a beverage that offers a quick and convenient energy boost for consumers.

**Caffeine Content:**

- Similar to coffee, most energy drinks contain high levels of caffeine, which of course can relax the *LES* allowing stomach acid to flow back into the esophagus, causing heartburn.

**Acidic Ingredients:**

- Like citrus drinks, some energy drinks may have high acidity levels due to ingredients like citric acid or other acidic additives. Increased acidity in the stomach can contribute to acid reflux.

**Carbonation:**

- Carbonated beverages, including certain energy drinks, release carbon dioxide gas, creating bubbles. This can increase pressure in the stomach, potentially pushing stomach acid into the esophagus and triggering reflux.

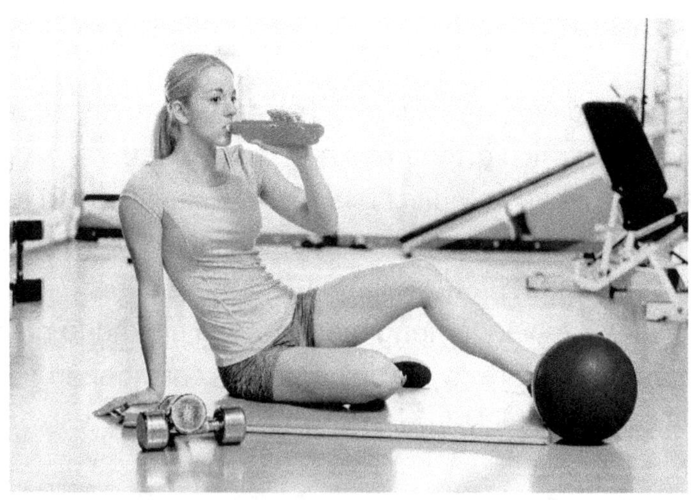

**Sugar and Additives:**

- Sugars and other additives found in energy drinks may contribute to digestive discomfort. High sugar content can lead to *Fermentation* in the stomach, producing gas that can push stomach contents upward.

**Dehydration:**

- Caffeine is a *diuretic*, meaning it can increase urine production and potentially lead to dehydration. Dehydration can affect the mucous lining of the *esophagus*, making it more susceptible to irritation from stomach acid.

**Timing of Consumption:**

- Consuming energy drinks close to bedtime may exacerbate acid reflux symptoms. The body naturally produces less saliva at night, which normally helps neutralize stomach acid. Additionally, lying down after consuming energy drinks can make it easier for stomach acid to flow back into the *esophagus*.

Individual sensitivity varies, and not everyone will experience acid reflux from consuming energy drinks. However, if you're prone to acid reflux or *GERD*, it's advisable to be cautious with energy drinks and consider alternative, less acidic beverage options to support digestive comfort.

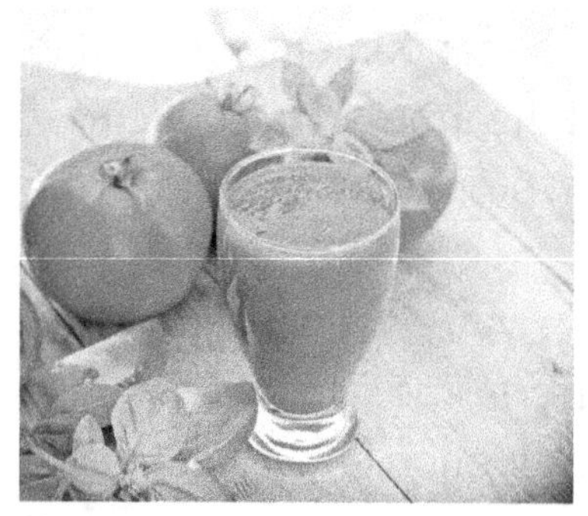 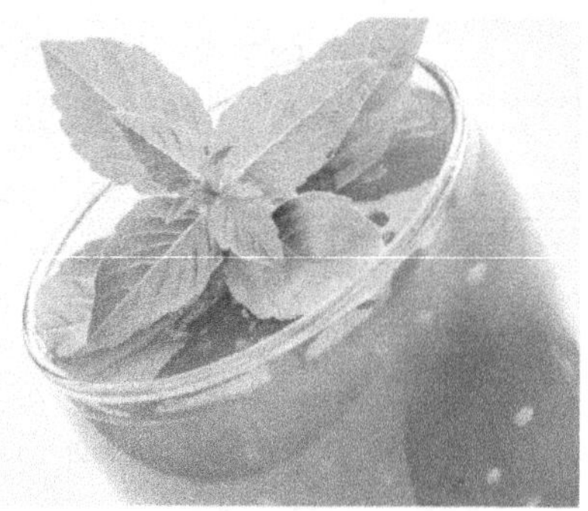

## Tomato Based Juices

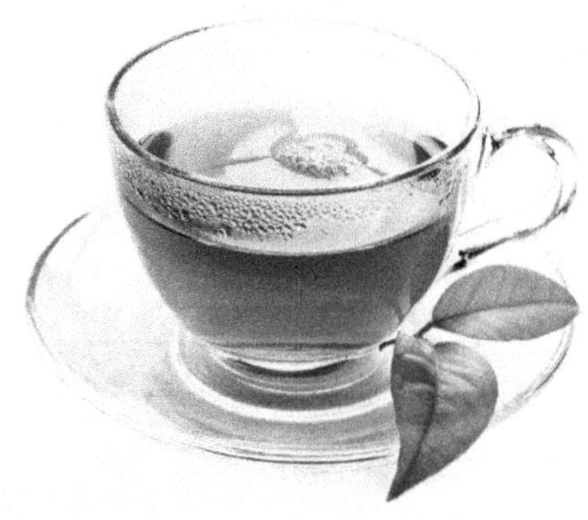 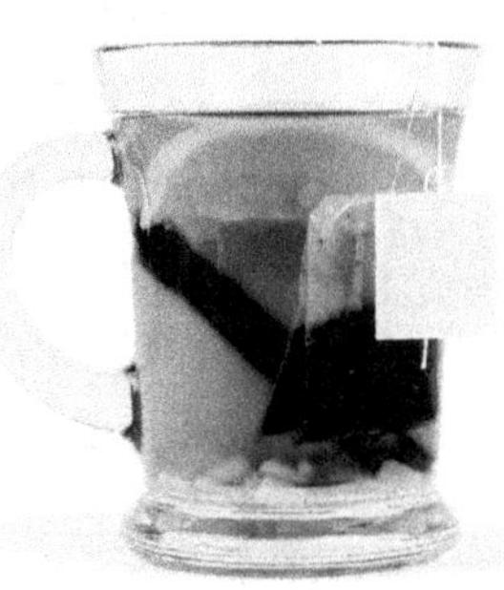

## Caffeinated Teas

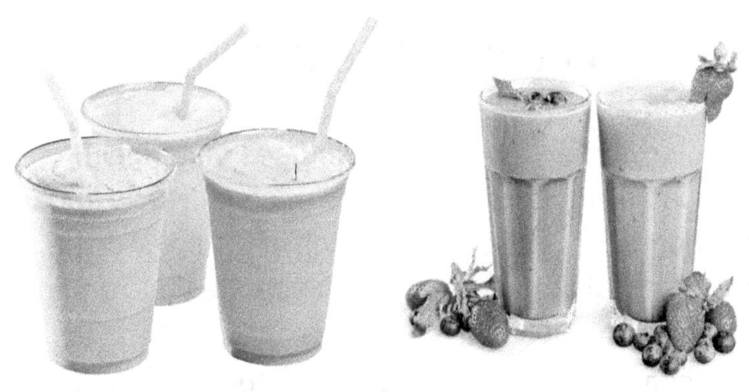

# Milkshakes and Smoothies

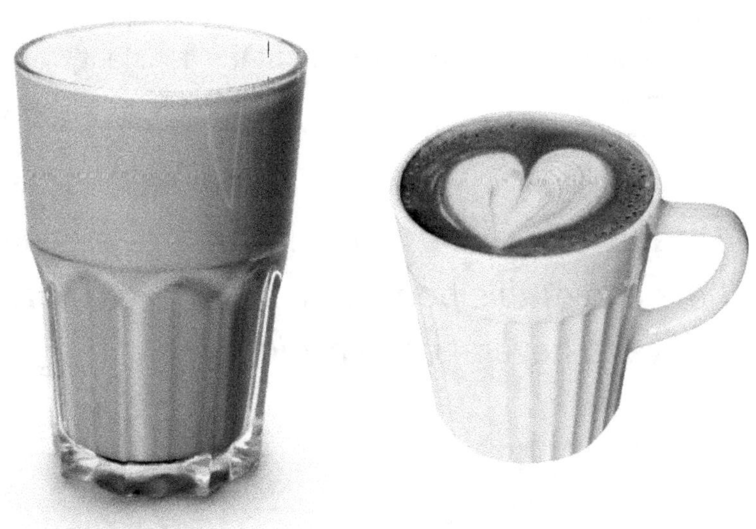

# Chocolate Milk & Cocoa

# To summarize food and beverage causes of heartburn

Avoiding certain foods and beverages that trigger heartburn is crucial to prevent the uncomfortable burning sensation in your chest. Foods high in fat, spicy dishes, caffeinated drinks, and acidic fruits irritate the stomach and *esophagus*, leading to heartburn. Alcohol and large meals can also relax the lower *esophageal sphincter*, making it easier for stomach acid to back up.

By understanding what triggers your heartburn and making dietary adjustments, you can significantly reduce discomfort. It's about taking care of your body and avoiding the foods and drinks that cause you pain, so you can feel better and enjoy life without the constant worry of heartburn.

** Please refer to the included quick reference at the end of this book for a list of even more foods and beverages to avoid.*

# SEVEN
## A Few Simple Adjustments

## Stay Upright After Meals

Pretty simple, but its importance cannot be overstated and is commonly overlooked. Maintaining an upright position after eating plays a crucial role in mitigating heartburn symptoms. When you sit or stand, gravity naturally aids in keeping the stomach's contents, including its acidic digestive juices, downward. This physical force helps prevent the backflow of acid into the *esophagus*, which is a primary cause of the burning sensation known as heartburn.

Lying down too soon after meals diminishes this gravitational advantage, making it easier for acidic fluids to travel back up, irritating the esophageal lining. By staying upright, you enhance the digestive process and ensure that the acids remain in the stomach where they belong, significantly reducing the risk of discomfort and promoting overall digestive health.

## Wear Loose-Fitting Clothes

Wearing loose-fitting clothes is a simple yet effective strategy to prevent heartburn. Tight clothing, especially around the waist and abdomen, can increase pressure on the stomach, pushing its contents upwards towards the esophagus. This pressure can force the *(LES)* to open inappropriately, allowing stomach acid to escape into the *esophagus* and cause the burning sensation associated with heartburn.

In contrast, loose clothing reduces this intra-abdominal pressure, minimizing the risk of acid reflux. By opting for garments that do not constrict the stomach area, you can help maintain a more natural digestive flow, thereby decreasing the likelihood of heartburn. This approach is particularly beneficial during activities such as eating or bending over, when pressure on the abdomen is naturally increased.

## Elevate the Head of Your Bed

The same principle as "staying upright after meals" applies to bedtime. Elevating the head of your bed is an effective strategy to reduce heartburn because it utilizes gravity to your advantage. By raising the bed's head, you create a slight incline from your head to your feet, which helps prevent stomach acid from traveling back up into the esophagus while you sleep. This positioning can significantly reduce the frequency and intensity of heartburn episodes, ensuring a more comfortable and restful night.

Additionally, this simple adjustment can improve overall digestion during the night, a time when the discomfort of heartburn can be particularly disruptive to sleep. It's a non-invasive, cost-effective solution that can complement other heartburn management strategies, offering relief to those suffering from *gastroesophageal reflux disease (GERD)* or occasional acid reflux.

There are several methods to elevate the head of your bed effectively to prevent heartburn, each varying in simplicity, cost, and adaptability:

1. **Bed Risers:** Place bed risers under the legs of the bed frame at the head of the bed. These are available in various heights, allowing you to choose how much you want to elevate the bed.

2. **Mattress Wedge:** A specially designed wedge can be placed between the mattress and the box spring or bed frame at the head of the bed. This raises the upper part of the mattress in a gradual slope.

3. **Foam Wedge Pillow:** Instead of adjusting the bed itself, you can use a foam wedge pillow to elevate your upper body. These pillows are designed to support the back and neck comfortably.

4. **Adjustable Bed:** If budget allows, an adjustable bed frame can be an excellent investment. These frames can be electronically controlled to raise the head of the bed to the desired angle, offering the most flexibility and comfort.

5. **DIY Methods:** For a quick and cost-effective solution, you can place sturdy objects like books, blocks of wood, or bricks under the legs of the bed frame at the head of the bed. Ensure that the bed is stable and secure to prevent any accidents.

6. **Extra Pillows:** Though not as effective as the other methods, using extra pillows to prop yourself up can provide temporary relief. However, this method can lead to neck or back pain due to improper alignment.

Choosing the right method depends on personal preference, the severity of heartburn, and whether you're looking for a temporary fix or a long-term solution. It's important to ensure that whatever method you choose provides stability and safety while sleeping.

# Reviewing Medications

Reviewing the medications you take is crucial because certain drugs can significantly contribute to heartburn by impacting the digestive system's normal functioning. Some medications will relax the *lower esophageal sphincter (LES)*. When the *LES* is weakened or relaxed, it cannot effectively block the acid, leading to acid reflux and the associated burning sensation. Examples of such medications include *Antihistamines*, certain antidepressants, and blood pressure medications.

Other drugs can irritate the *esophagus* directly or increase acid production in the stomach, exacerbating heartburn symptoms. For instance, aspirin and other **non-steroidal anti-inflammatory drugs (NSAIDs)** can irritate the stomach and esophageal lining, while some supplements and vitamins, like iron or potassium, can do the same. Even medications intended to improve health can have unintended side effects that affect the digestive tract.

Therefore, it's important to review all medications, including over-the-counter drugs and supplements, with a healthcare provider. They can assess the risk of heartburn in relation to your medication regimen and might suggest alternatives or adjustments to mitigate these effects. This review process is a proactive step in managing and preventing heartburn, ensuring that treatment for one condition does not detrimentally impact another.

# EIGHT

# Alternative (Holistic) Therapies

## Herbal Remedies:

**<u>Swedish Bitters:</u>** *Swedish Bitters*, a traditional herbal tonic made from a mixture of herbs soaked in alcohol, has been used for centuries as a remedy for a variety of ailments, including digestive issues such as heartburn. The formula is believed to have originated in the 18th century and was popularized by a Swedish physician named Dr. Claus Samst. The formulation of Swedish Bitters can vary, but it typically includes herbs such as aloe, rhubarb, senna, myrrh, and saffron, among others. These herbs are known for their digestive, anti-inflammatory, and healing properties, which can contribute to the prevention and alleviation of heartburn symptoms.

Heartburn can be triggered by factors such as overeating, stress, or certain foods and beverages. The complex blend of herbs in Swedish Bitters works synergistically to address various aspects of digestive health that can contribute to heartburn.

Firstly, Swedish Bitters is believed to stimulate the production of digestive enzymes and saliva, which can help in the more efficient breakdown and assimilation of food. This reduces the likelihood of indigestion and the occurrence of heartburn, as food is less likely to linger in the stomach and provoke acid reflux. Additionally, the tonic can increase *bile* production, aiding in the digestion of fats that can otherwise slow down the digestive process and contribute to heartburn symptoms.

Some herbs in Swedish Bitters, such as myrrh and aloe, have anti-inflammatory properties that can soothe the gastrointestinal tract, reducing inflammation and irritation caused by stomach acid in the *esophagus*. This can provide relief from the discomfort associated with heartburn.

Moreover, Swedish Bitters is thought to have a tonic effect on the stomach and the entire digestive system, strengthening the function of these organs over time. By improving overall digestive health, Swedish Bitters can help prevent the conditions that lead to heartburn. It's also believed to improve the tone of the *lower esophageal sphincter (LES)*, the muscle that separates the stomach from the esophagus. A stronger *LES* is less likely to allow stomach acid to reflux into the *esophagus*, thus preventing heartburn.

However, it's important to approach the use of Swedish Bitters with caution. While it can be beneficial for preventing heartburn, it's not suitable for everyone. The alcohol content and certain herbs like senna, which has a laxative effect, may not be appropriate for individuals with certain health conditions, pregnant or breastfeeding women, or those taking specific medications. It's essential to consult with a healthcare professional before starting any new remedy, including Swedish Bitters, to ensure it's safe and appropriate for your specific health situation.

In conclusion, Swedish Bitters can offer a natural and holistic approach to preventing heartburn through its blend of digestive-stimulating, anti-inflammatory, and tonic herbs. By supporting digestive health and improving the function of the digestive system, it can help mitigate the factors that contribute to heartburn, providing relief and improving overall well-being.

## Ginger: *Ginger*, a root herb known for its strong, spicy flavor and aromatic qualities, has been used for centuries in various traditional medicine systems worldwide to treat a myriad of health conditions, including digestive issues like heartburn. The natural properties of ginger can help prevent and alleviate these symptoms through several mechanisms.

Firstly, ginger possesses potent anti-inflammatory properties that can soothe the gastrointestinal tract, reducing the inflammation and irritation caused by acid reflux. This anti-inflammatory effect is largely attributed to *gingerols*, the main bioactive compounds in ginger, which have been shown to inhibit the synthesis of pro-inflammatory *cytokines* in the gut, thus reducing inflammation and potentially preventing the onset of heartburn.

Additionally, ginger is known to promote the movement of food and liquids through the digestive system more efficiently. This *prokinetic* effect can prevent the accumulation of food and stomach acid that might otherwise back up into the *esophagus*, triggering heartburn. By enhancing gastric motility, ginger helps ensure that stomach contents are emptied into the small intestine more rapidly, reducing the risk of acid reflux.

Ginger also has a mild **Anti–Emetic Effect**, which can help reduce nausea and discomfort often associated with digestive disturbances, including those that can lead to heartburn. This property makes ginger a beneficial adjunct in managing gastrointestinal symptoms and improving overall digestive health.

Despite its benefits, ginger should be used in moderation. Excessive consumption can lead to digestive discomfort for some individuals. It's also important for individuals with gallstones, bleeding disorders, or those on blood thinners to consult a healthcare professional before incorporating high doses of ginger into their diet, as it may interact with certain medical conditions and medications.

The use of ginger can serve as a natural and effective way to prevent heartburn. Its anti-inflammatory, *prokinetic*, and *antiemetic* properties work together to improve digestive health, alleviate gastrointestinal irritation, and reduce the frequency and severity of heartburn episodes.

## **Chamomile Tea:** *Chamomile Tea* is widely recognized for its calming and soothing properties, making it a popular herbal remedy for various ailments, including the prevention of heartburn. This gentle tea is made from the dried flowers of the chamomile plant, which contain several *bioactive* compounds, such as *flavonoids* and **terpenoids**, known for their therapeutic effects. One of the primary ways chamomile tea can help prevent heartburn is through its anti-inflammatory properties, which may reduce the inflammation in the *gastrointestinal tract* that can contribute to acid reflux and the discomfort of heartburn.

Additionally, chamomile tea has a mild sedative effect that can relax the muscles of the upper digestive tract, helping to prevent spasms and reduce the likelihood of stomach acid escaping into the *esophagus*. This relaxation can also extend to the *lower esophageal sphincter (LES)*, ensuring it closes properly after food passes through, which is crucial in preventing reflux.

Moreover, chamomile tea is believed to balance stomach acid levels and aid in overall digestion, further minimizing the risk of heartburn. Its gentle nature makes it a suitable option for many, including those looking for a natural way to ease digestive discomfort.

Drinking chamomile tea in moderation before or after meals can be a simple, effective way to incorporate its benefits into a heartburn prevention regimen. However, as with any herbal remedy, it's wise to consult with a healthcare provider, especially for those with allergies to plants in the daisy family, pregnant women, or individuals on medication, to ensure it's appropriate for their health situation.

## **Licorice:** *Licorice*, derived from the root of the plant *Glycyrrhiza Glabra*, has been traditionally used for various health issues, including gastrointestinal problems like heartburn. The active compound in licorice, *glycyrrhizin*, has anti-inflammatory and soothing properties that may help in preventing and alleviating heartburn symptoms.

The mechanism behind licorice's beneficial effects involves its ability to enhance the mucosal defense of the *gastrointestinal tract*. This is achieved by increasing the production of mucin, a key component of the protective mucus layer that lines the stomach and *esophagus*. This enhanced mucosal defense helps to prevent the irritation and inflammation caused by stomach acids. Additionally, licorice has been found to stimulate the secretion of gastric mucus, which further aids in protecting the esophageal and stomach lining from acid damage.

*Deglycyrrhizinated licorice (DGL)* is a form of licorice that has had the *glycyrrhizin* removed to avoid potential side effects such as increased blood pressure and water retention associated with glycyrrhizin. DGL retains the beneficial properties of licorice for gastrointestinal health without the associated risks, making it a safer option for those looking to manage heartburn symptoms.

It's important to note that while licorice can be effective in preventing heartburn, it should be used judiciously. High doses or long-term use can lead to adverse effects. Therefore, individuals interested in using licorice for heartburn should consider consulting a healthcare professional, especially if they have existing health conditions or are taking other medications. This ensures that licorice is used safely and effectively as part of a holistic approach to managing heartburn.

## **Marshmallow Root:** *Marshmallow Root,*

derived from the ***Althaea Officinalis Plant,*** has been utilized in traditional herbal medicine for centuries, serving as a natural remedy for various ailments, especially those related to the digestive system, such as heartburn. The therapeutic properties of marshmallow root can help prevent and alleviate heartburn through several key actions.

The primary mechanism by which marshmallow root aids in preventing heartburn is its high *mucilage* content. *Mucilage* is a slippery, gel-like substance that, when mixed with water, forms a soothing protective layer on the lining of the digestive tract. This layer acts as a barrier against stomach acid, preventing it from irritating the *esophagus* and thereby reducing the occurrence of heartburn. The *mucilage* not only shields the esophageal lining from acid damage but also promotes healing of any existing irritation or inflammation, offering relief from discomfort.

Moreover, marshmallow root has anti-inflammatory properties that further support its role in soothing irritated mucous membranes within the digestive tract. By reducing inflammation, it helps to alleviate the symptoms associated with acid reflux, such as pain and discomfort.

In addition to its protective and anti-inflammatory effects, marshmallow root can also help improve digestive health overall. It supports proper digestion by encouraging a healthy balance of gut flora and may enhance the body's natural digestive processes, reducing the likelihood of acid reflux and heartburn.

It's important to note that while marshmallow root can be an effective natural remedy for preventing heartburn, individuals should consult with a healthcare provider before starting any new treatment, especially those with pre-existing health conditions or those taking other medications, to avoid potential interactions. Marshmallow root can be consumed in various forms, including teas, capsules, or extracts, offering a versatile and gentle option for those seeking natural support for digestive health and the prevention of heartburn.

**Slippery Elm:** *Slippery Elm*, derived from the inner bark of the **Ulmus Rubra Tree**, is a traditional herbal remedy known for its soothing and healing properties, especially in the digestive system. Its effectiveness in preventing heartburn stems from the *mucilage* it contains—a gel-like substance that becomes a slick gel when mixed with water. This *mucilage* coats and protects the mucous membranes lining the *esophagus* and stomach, thereby providing relief from heartburn and other forms of gastrointestinal discomfort.

When consumed, Slippery Elm's *mucilage* forms a protective barrier against the corrosive effects of stomach acid on the *esophagus*. This barrier not only prevents the irritation and burning sensation often experienced with acid reflux but also promotes healing in areas that have been damaged or inflamed. By enhancing the body's natural mucosal defenses, Slippery Elm helps to maintain a healthy, well-lubricated digestive tract, which is less susceptible to the damaging effects of acid reflux.

Moreover, Slippery Elm can improve digestion by stimulating nerve endings in the *gastrointestinal tract*, which in turn can help to reduce the occurrence of heartburn. Its soothing properties also extend to overall digestive health by promoting the secretion of mucus, which protects the *gastrointestinal tract* and aids in the smooth passage of food through the digestive system, reducing the likelihood of acid buildup and reflux.

Given its gentle nature, Slippery Elm is considered safe for most people and can be taken in various forms, such as teas, capsules, or powders. However, individuals with specific health conditions or those taking prescription medications should consult a healthcare professional before incorporating Slippery Elm into their regimen, to ensure it complements their overall health strategy effectively.

**<u>Aloe Vera Juice:</u>** *Aloe Vera Juice*, derived from the inner leaf gel of the ***Aloe Vera plant***, has long been celebrated for its soothing and healing properties, particularly in relation to digestive health. Its use in preventing heartburn is attributed to several key mechanisms that support the *gastrointestinal tract's* overall well-being.

The anti-inflammatory properties of Aloe Vera Juice are crucial in managing heartburn symptoms. By reducing inflammation in the *esophagus* and stomach, Aloe Vera Juice can help soothe irritation caused by the reflux of stomach acid. This not only alleviates the discomfort associated with heartburn but also assists in healing the damaged mucosal lining, providing a protective effect against further acid exposure.

Aloe Vera Juice also has a mild laxative effect, which can aid in improving digestion and ensuring smoother bowel movements. This aspect is beneficial as it prevents the buildup of pressure in the stomach, a common contributor to acid reflux. By enhancing digestive efficiency and reducing stomach pressure, Aloe Vera Juice can minimize the instances of acid backing up into the *esophagus*, thereby preventing heartburn episodes.

Additionally, Aloe Vera Juice is believed to balance stomach acid levels. By maintaining a healthy acid balance, it can prevent the harsh effects of excessive stomach acid, which is often a direct cause of heartburn.

Despite its benefits, it's important for individuals considering Aloe Vera Juice for heartburn to choose products free from aloin, a compound with potent laxative effects, and to consult with a healthcare professional. This ensures the juice's compatibility with their health profile and avoids potential side effects, making Aloe Vera Juice a safe and effective remedy for preventing heartburn.

## Fennel: *Fennel*, a flavorful herb native to the Mediterranean, has been utilized for centuries in traditional medicine for its digestive benefits. Recognized by its licorice-like taste, fennel seeds are particularly valued for their ability to alleviate digestive problems, including heartburn. Fennel's unique properties can help prevent this discomfort through several mechanisms, making it a natural and effective remedy.

One of the primary ways fennel aids in preventing heartburn is through its **antispasmodic properties**. These properties allow fennel to relax the muscles in the *gastrointestinal tract*, reducing spasms that can push stomach acid into the *esophagus*. By calming the stomach and digestive muscles, fennel helps to prevent the reflux of stomach contents, thereby mitigating the risk of heartburn.

Additionally, fennel seeds contain compounds like **anethole**, **fenchone**, and **estragole**, which have been found to stimulate digestion and reduce inflammation in the digestive tract. This not only helps in soothing the stomach lining but also promotes a more efficient digestion process, reducing the likelihood of acid buildup and reflux.

Fennel also acts as a natural *carminative*, meaning it aids in the expulsion of gas from the stomach and intestines. This property is beneficial in preventing the uncomfortable bloating that can increase intra-abdominal pressure, a common trigger for acid reflux. By reducing gas and bloating, fennel helps maintain a healthy pressure balance in the stomach, thus preventing the conditions that lead to heartburn.

Moreover, fennel seeds are a rich source of dietary fiber, which supports healthy digestion and regular bowel movements. This fiber content helps to absorb stomach acids and promotes a healthy gut environment, further contributing to the prevention of heartburn.

To incorporate fennel into the diet for its heartburn-preventing benefits, one can chew on fennel seeds after meals, brew them into a soothing tea, or include fennel bulbs in salads and dishes. While fennel is generally safe for consumption, individuals with specific health conditions or allergies should consult a healthcare provider before adding it to their dietary regimen.

# Dietary Supplements:

Dietary supplements can serve as a helpful addition in managing and reducing heartburn symptoms by supporting digestive health, strengthening the gastrointestinal lining, and balancing stomach acid. Here are a few supplements that are commonly used for this purpose.

It's important to approach the use of dietary supplements with caution and consult with a healthcare provider before starting any new supplement, especially for individuals with existing health conditions or those taking other medications. Supplements can interact with medications and may not be suitable for everyone.

## **Magnesium:** *Magnesium*, a vital mineral for many bodily functions, plays a significant role in digestive health and can be particularly beneficial in preventing heartburn. The efficacy of *magnesium* in preventing heartburn is linked to its ability to improve digestive function and regulate muscle relaxation within the *gastrointestinal tract*.

One of the primary ways magnesium aids in preventing heartburn is through its role in muscle relaxation. Magnesium helps to relax the *LES* when it needs to open, ensuring it functions correctly. However, it's important that the *LES* remains tight enough to prevent acid reflux. Magnesium's ability to balance muscle relaxation and contraction can help maintain optimal *LES* function, reducing the likelihood of heartburn.

Magnesium also contributes to overall digestive health by supporting the movement of food through the digestive tract. It stimulates *peristalsis*, the series of wave-like muscle contractions that move food along the digestive tract, ensuring efficient digestion and reducing the risk of stomach acid building up and leading to heartburn.

Furthermore, magnesium is involved in more than 300 *enzymatic reactions* in the body, including those necessary for energy production and nutrient metabolism. By facilitating these processes, magnesium can help ensure that the digestive system has the energy it needs to function optimally, reducing the occurrence of digestive disturbances like heartburn.

In addition to its direct benefits on the digestive system, magnesium can also counteract excess acidity in the stomach. While not a traditional antacid, magnesium can neutralize stomach acid to a certain extent, providing temporary relief from heartburn symptoms.

Magnesium's effectiveness in preventing heartburn is also linked to its ability to combat stress, a common trigger for acid reflux. Magnesium has a calming effect on the nervous system, which can help reduce stress levels and, consequently, the likelihood of stress-induced heartburn.

Despite these benefits, it's important to use magnesium supplements responsibly. Excessive magnesium intake, especially from supplements, can lead to adverse effects, including diarrhea, which can exacerbate heartburn in some cases. The recommended approach is to obtain magnesium from a balanced diet rich in magnesium-containing foods, such as leafy green vegetables, nuts, seeds, and whole grains. For those considering magnesium supplements, consulting with a healthcare provider is essential to determine the appropriate dosage and ensure it does not interact with other medications or health conditions.

In summary, magnesium plays a multifaceted role in preventing heartburn, from supporting *LES* function and promoting digestive health to balancing stomach acid and reducing stress. Its comprehensive impact on the body underscores the importance of maintaining adequate magnesium levels for overall health and well-being.

## **Melatonin:** *Melatonin*, a hormone primarily

known for its role in regulating sleep-wake cycles, has emerged as a surprising ally in the prevention of heartburn and *gastroesophageal reflux disease (GERD)*. Beyond its sleep-regulating functions, melatonin exhibits properties that can significantly impact digestive health, particularly in protecting the *esophagus* from the corrosive effects of stomach acid.

The connection between melatonin and heartburn prevention is multifaceted. One of the primary mechanisms involves melatonin's ability to strengthen the *(LES)*. When the *LES* is weakened or relaxes inappropriately, it allows acid to escape the stomach, leading to heartburn. Melatonin can improve the tone and function of the *LES*, reducing the likelihood of acid reflux and, consequently, heartburn.

Additionally, melatonin is believed to have a protective effect on the **gastrointestinal mucosa**—the lining of the digestive tract. It does this by enhancing the production of **prostaglandins**, substances that promote mucosal defense mechanisms. This increased protection can prevent the irritation and damage caused by stomach acids, further contributing to the prevention of heartburn.

Melatonin also possesses **antioxidant properties**, which play a role in reducing inflammation in the *gastrointestinal tract*. Inflammation can exacerbate heartburn symptoms by making the esophagus more sensitive to acid exposure. By mitigating inflammation, melatonin can alleviate the discomfort associated with heartburn.

Research has suggested that melatonin may work synergistically with other antioxidants and vitamins, such as vitamin B6, to provide a comprehensive approach to preventing heartburn. This combination not only strengthens the *LES* and mucosal defenses but also promotes overall digestive health, reducing the incidence and severity of heartburn episodes.

Interestingly, melatonin's role in preventing heartburn extends to its influence on the nervous system. Stress and anxiety can exacerbate heartburn symptoms by increasing stomach acid production and sensitivity to pain. As a natural relaxant, melatonin can help reduce stress levels, thereby indirectly contributing to the prevention of heartburn.

Despite these promising attributes, it's important to approach the use of melatonin with caution. While short-term use is generally considered safe for most individuals, long-term effects are still not fully understood. Additionally, melatonin can interact with various medications and conditions, making it crucial for individuals to consult with a healthcare professional before starting melatonin supplements, especially if they are already managing other health issues or taking prescription drugs.

In conclusion, the use of melatonin as a preventive measure against heartburn represents an innovative and holistic approach. By strengthening the *LES*, enhancing mucosal protection, reducing inflammation, and managing stress, melatonin addresses multiple facets of heartburn. However, as with any supplement, a balanced diet, healthy lifestyle choices, and medical guidance are essential components of an effective heartburn prevention strategy.

## **<u>Zinc Carnosine:</u>** *Zinc Carnosine*, a *chelated compound* consisting of zinc and carnosine, has garnered attention for its potential benefits in gastrointestinal health, specifically in the prevention and management of heartburn. The unique properties of Zinc Carnosine offer a promising approach to mitigate this common and uncomfortable condition.

At the cellular level, Zinc Carnosine has been shown to strengthen the mucosal lining of the stomach, offering a protective barrier against the corrosive nature of stomach acid. This protective effect not only helps to prevent the onset of heartburn but also promotes the healing of existing damage to the esophageal lining. Zinc, an essential mineral, plays a crucial role in tissue repair and the maintenance of healthy cells. When combined with carnosine, a *dipeptide* with *antioxidant properties*, the compound enhances the defense against *oxidative stress*, which is often a contributing factor to the deterioration of the gastrointestinal lining.

Zinc Carnosine also has been reported to stabilize the gastric mucosal barrier and regulate gastric acid secretion. By doing so, it addresses two critical factors in the development of heartburn: the integrity of the mucosal lining and the amount of acid produced by the stomach. This dual action makes Zinc Carnosine a comprehensive solution for managing symptoms related to acid reflux.

Clinical studies have supported the efficacy of Zinc Carnosine in improving gastrointestinal health. Patients receiving Zinc Carnosine supplementation have shown significant improvement in symptoms associated with heartburn, including reduced frequency and severity of episodes. This evidence suggests that Zinc Carnosine not only provides symptomatic relief but may also contribute to the long-term health of the *gastrointestinal tract*.

In addition to its protective and healing properties, Zinc Carnosine's safety profile makes it a favorable option for many individuals. Unlike some traditional heartburn medications that may have adverse effects or interact with other medications, Zinc Carnosine offers a natural, gentle alternative that can be used as part of a comprehensive approach to managing gastrointestinal health.

In conclusion, Zinc Carnosine presents a promising and multifaceted approach to preventing and managing heartburn. Its unique ability to strengthen the mucosal lining, regulate acid secretion, and protect against oxidative stress addresses the root causes of heartburn, offering not just symptomatic relief but also contributing to the overall health of the gastrointestinal system. As research continues to unfold, Zinc Carnosine may become an increasingly popular choice for those seeking natural and effective ways to maintain their digestive health.

# Apple Cider Vinegar: *Apple Cider Vinegar*

*(ACV)* has been touted as a natural remedy for a variety of health issues, including heartburn. Despite its acidic nature, *ACV* is believed to help prevent heartburn by balancing stomach acidity levels and improving digestion.

The mechanism by which ACV may help prevent heartburn is multifaceted. Firstly, it is thought that ACV can increase the acidity of the stomach when it is too low. A properly acidic environment in the stomach is crucial for the digestion of food and the absorption of nutrients. When stomach acid is insufficient, digestion is impaired, leading to food sitting in the stomach for longer than necessary, which can increase the risk of acid reflux. By enhancing stomach acidity, ACV helps ensure efficient digestion and reduces the likelihood of heartburn.

Additionally, ACV is rich in **enzymes** and **probiotics** due to the fermentation process it undergoes. These components are believed to aid in digestion and support a healthy *gut microbiome*, further reducing the occurrence of digestive discomfort and heartburn. A well-balanced *gut flora* is essential for optimal digestive health, as it helps break down food, absorbs nutrients, and keeps harmful bacteria in check.

It's important to note, however, that the use of ACV for preventing heartburn should be approached with caution. Due to its acidic nature, it should be diluted in water before consumption to avoid damaging tooth enamel or irritating the *esophagus*. While many individuals report relief from heartburn symptoms with ACV, its effectiveness can vary, and it may not be suitable for everyone, particularly those with a history of esophageal erosion or other digestive disorders.

In summary, Apple Cider Vinegar may offer a natural way to prevent heartburn by improving stomach acidity, enhancing digestion, and supporting gut health. However, its use should be individualized, and those with existing digestive issues should consult with a healthcare professional before incorporating ACV into their regimen.

# Acupuncture:

*Acupuncture*, an ancient Chinese medical practice, has been utilized for thousands of years to treat a variety of ailments, including digestive issues such as heartburn. Despite the prevalence of pharmaceutical remedies for heartburn, many individuals seek alternative treatments like *acupuncture* to manage their symptoms, aiming for a holistic approach to their health.

Acupuncture involves the insertion of thin needles into specific points on the body, known as acupuncture points, to restore balance and promote the body's natural healing processes. According to Traditional Chinese Medicine (TCM), heartburn is often a sign of an imbalance in the body's energy flow, or **Qi**, particularly in the stomach or **spleen meridians**. Acupuncture aims to correct these imbalances, thereby alleviating symptoms of heartburn.

The theoretical basis of acupuncture in treating heartburn centers on its ability to regulate the flow of Qi and restore harmony within the body's internal organs. Practitioners believe that by targeting specific acupuncture points related to the digestive system, they can strengthen the stomach and spleen, enhance digestive functions, and prevent the improper ascent of stomach acid.

Scientific research offers insights into how acupuncture can be effective in preventing heartburn. Studies suggest that acupuncture can stimulate the nervous system, leading to the release of neurotransmitters and hormones that can influence **gastric secretion**, enhance **intestinal motility**, and improve overall gut health. These physiological changes can reduce gastric acidity and increase the efficiency of the digestive process, thus reducing the likelihood of acid reflux.

Moreover, acupuncture is thought to increase the *lower esophageal sphincter (LES)* tone. By strengthening the

*LES*, acupuncture can provide a mechanical barrier to acid reflux, thereby preventing heartburn.

Acupuncture also addresses stress, which is a known trigger for heartburn. Stress can exacerbate symptoms of acid reflux by increasing stomach acid production and compromising the digestive process. Acupuncture is renowned for its ability to induce relaxation and reduce stress levels. By calming the mind and reducing stress, acupuncture can indirectly prevent the occurrence of heartburn by mitigating one of its common triggers.

Furthermore, acupuncture promotes holistic well-being by encouraging patients to adopt healthier lifestyles. Practitioners often provide dietary advice and recommend specific exercises along with acupuncture treatment to enhance digestive health and prevent heartburn. Such comprehensive care can lead to long-term improvements in gastrointestinal function and a reduction in heartburn episodes.

While acupuncture offers a promising alternative to conventional treatments for heartburn, it is important to approach this therapy with informed expectations. The effectiveness of acupuncture can vary among individuals, and its benefits are often maximized when combined with other lifestyle modifications, such as dietary changes and stress management techniques. It is crucial to seek treatment from a licensed and experienced acupuncturist to ensure safety and efficacy.

In conclusion, acupuncture represents a valuable and holistic approach to preventing heartburn. By targeting specific acupuncture points related to the digestive system, it aims to restore the balance of *Qi*, strengthen the digestive organs, enhance the function of the *LES*, and alleviate stress. Through these mechanisms, it's possible acupuncture can improve digestive health and prevent the uncomfortable symptoms of heartburn. As part of a broader strategy that includes dietary and lifestyle adjustments, acupuncture can provide a natural and effective solution for those seeking to manage their heartburn symptoms without relying solely on medication.

Its growing popularity as an alternative treatment underscores the desire for holistic approaches to health care, emphasizing the importance of treating the body as an interconnected system

# Stress Reduction Techniques:

Heartburn, often triggered or exacerbated by stress, can be significantly managed through various stress reduction techniques. Stress affects the body in multiple ways, including increasing stomach acid production and causing muscle tension, which can worsen heartburn symptoms. Implementing stress reduction strategies can help mitigate these effects and improve overall well-being. Here are some effective techniques which may help some readers to reduce stress and potentially decrease the frequency and severity of heartburn episodes:

## **Deep Breathing Exercises:** Deep breathing exercises are a simple yet effective method to prevent heartburn, a symptom often exacerbated by stress and anxiety. These exercises work by activating the *parasympathetic nervous system*, which promotes a state of relaxation and can help mitigate the physiological effects of stress that contribute to acid reflux and heartburn. When stressed, individuals may experience an increase in stomach acid production and a tightening of muscles, including those around the stomach and *esophagus*, potentially worsening heartburn symptoms.

Practicing deep breathing exercises encourages the relaxation of the body's muscles, reducing tension in the *gastrointestinal tract*. This relaxation can help prevent the spasms that force stomach acid back into the *esophagus*, thereby reducing the occurrence of heartburn. Moreover, deep breathing can decrease overall stress levels, which is beneficial since stress is a known trigger for acid reflux.

One popular deep breathing technique that can be particularly effective in managing heartburn is **diaphragmatic breathing**. This involves focusing on breathing deeply into the diaphragm rather than shallowly into the chest, facilitating more efficient oxygen exchange and further promoting relaxation throughout the body. By regularly practicing *diaphragmatic breathing* or other deep breathing exercises, individuals can enhance their digestive function, lessen the likelihood of acid reflux episodes, and thereby prevent the discomfort associated with heartburn.

Incorporating deep breathing exercises into daily routines can be a proactive and natural approach to managing heartburn. These exercises not only offer immediate relief from stress but also serve as a preventative measure against the development of heartburn, contributing to improved gastrointestinal health and overall well-being.

# Mindfulness and Meditation: This

practice has emerged as a powerful strategy for managing stress and improving overall health, including the prevention of heartburn. The practice of mindfulness and meditation can directly address the stress component, thereby reducing the frequency and severity of heartburn episodes.

*Mindfulness*, (the act of being fully present and engaged in the moment without judgment), helps individuals become more aware of their body's signals and responses to stress. This heightened awareness can lead to a better understanding of the triggers that exacerbate heartburn, such as certain foods, eating habits, or emotional stressors. By recognizing these triggers, individuals can take proactive steps to avoid them, thereby preventing heartburn.

*Meditation*, particularly mindfulness meditation, involves focusing the mind on a particular object, thought, or activity to train attention and awareness. This practice can significantly reduce stress levels by inducing a state of relaxation and calm. Stress is known to affect the digestive system by increasing stomach acid production and causing muscle tension, both of which can lead to heartburn. By reducing stress through meditation, individuals can mitigate these physiological responses, decrease stomach acid production, and relax the muscles around the stomach and *esophagus*, preventing acid reflux.

Regular meditation practice can improve the body's response to stress over time, leading to long-term benefits for managing heartburn. It can enhance the regulation of the nervous system, improve digestive function, and strengthen the mind-body connection, fostering a greater sense of well-being and resilience against stress-induced heartburn.

Incorporating this technique into daily routines does not require extensive time commitments; even short periods of practice can be beneficial. By dedicating time to these practices, it is possible that some individuals can develop more effective coping mechanisms for stress, reduce their risk of heartburn, and enhance their overall quality of life.

## **Progressive Muscle Relaxation (PMR):**

*Progressive Muscle Relaxation (PMR)* is a stress-reduction technique that can be particularly effective in preventing heartburn, a condition often triggered or exacerbated by stress and tension. PMR involves systematically tensing and then relaxing different muscle groups throughout the body, which can lead to a profound state of physical relaxation. This method not only helps in alleviating stress but also directly impacts the physiological factors associated with heartburn.

By promoting overall muscle relaxation, PMR can reduce tension in the *gastrointestinal tract*, including the muscles around the stomach and *lower esophageal sphincter (LES)*. Stress and tension can weaken this muscle's ability to function correctly, leading to acid reflux and heartburn. Through the relaxation induced by PMR, the *LES* can maintain a tighter seal, thereby reducing the likelihood of acid reflux.

Regular practice of PMR can provide not only immediate relief from stress but also long-term benefits in reducing the frequency and severity of heartburn episodes, offering a natural and effective management strategy.

## **Yoga:** *Yoga*, an ancient practice that combines physical postures, breathing exercises, and meditation, offers a holistic approach to preventing and managing heartburn. Heartburn is often exacerbated by factors such as stress, obesity, and poor posture. *Yoga* addresses these underlying issues, providing a natural and effective way to prevent heartburn by enhancing physical health, reducing stress, and improving digestive function.

**Physical Benefits -** Yoga postures (*asanas*) can directly influence the physical factors contributing to heartburn. Certain asanas strengthen the abdominal and pelvic muscles, supporting the digestive organs and improving the efficiency of the *gastrointestinal tract*. This increased muscle tone can help prevent the excessive backward flow of stomach acid into the *esophagus*. Yoga also promotes weight loss and reduces abdominal fat, a known risk factor for acid reflux, by increasing overall physical activity and enhancing metabolic rate.

**Stress Reduction -** Stress is a significant trigger for heartburn, as it can increase stomach acid production and lead to muscle tension, including in the digestive tract. Yoga's emphasis on deep, controlled breathing and mindfulness meditation is particularly effective in activating the *parasympathetic nervous system*, which induces a state of relaxation and stress relief. By lowering stress levels, yoga can reduce the likelihood of stress-induced acid reflux episodes.

**Improved Posture -** Poor posture, especially while sitting or standing, can compress the abdomen and exacerbate heartburn symptoms. Yoga postures encourage alignment and strengthen the core muscles, leading to improved posture both on and off the mat. This alleviation of abdominal pressure can prevent the stomach contents from pushing upwards into the *esophagus*, thereby reducing the risk of acid reflux.

**Enhancing Digestive Function -** Yoga stimulates the digestive system, helping to facilitate smoother digestion and prevent issues like heartburn. Certain yoga poses, such as twisting poses, gently massage the internal organs, including the stomach and intestines, promoting the movement of food and aiding in the elimination of waste. This can prevent the buildup of stomach acid and ensure that the digestive process functions more efficiently.

## Selective Asanas for Heartburn Prevention -

While yoga, in general, can be beneficial for preventing heartburn, certain poses are particularly effective:

- *Vajrasana* (Thunderbolt Pose): Sitting on the heels with a straight spine after meals can aid in digestion and prevent acid reflux.
- *Ardha Matsyendrasana* (Half Spinal Twist): This twisting pose can massage abdominal organs, stimulating digestion and relieving symptoms of acid reflux.
- *Marjariasana* (Cat-Cow Stretch): The alternation between these two poses promotes flexibility in the spine and massages the digestive organs, enhancing digestive function.
- *Uttana Shishosana* (Extended Puppy Pose): This pose helps in stretching the abdomen, relieving stress, and encouraging proper digestion.

**Considerations and Cautions -** While yoga offers many benefits for preventing heartburn, it's important to practice with awareness and caution. Not all yoga poses are suitable for individuals experiencing heartburn. Inverted poses or those that involve lying down immediately after eating might worsen symptoms for some people. It's recommended to practice yoga on an empty stomach or several hours after a meal and to consult with a yoga instructor experienced in addressing digestive issues.

## Conclusion

Yoga presents a comprehensive approach to preventing heartburn by addressing the physical, emotional, and functional aspects contributing to acid reflux. Its practice promotes a stronger, more flexible body, reduces stress, improves posture, and enhances digestive health. Incorporating yoga into one's lifestyle not only offers a natural remedy for heartburn but also contributes to overall well-being and health.

As with any exercise regimen, it's essential to listen to your body and adapt practices to suit individual needs and conditions, potentially under the guidance of healthcare and yoga professionals. Through regular and mindful yoga practice, individuals can achieve significant relief from heartburn and improve their quality of life.

## <u>Regular Exercise:</u> Regular Exercise is a

cornerstone of good health, offering myriad benefits that extend to the prevention and management of heartburn, or acid reflux. The relationship between physical activity and heartburn is multifaceted, involving weight management, stress reduction, and the strengthening of the digestive system, each contributing to the mitigation of heartburn symptoms.

**Weight Management -** Weight Management is one of the most significant benefits of regular exercise in weight management. Excess weight, particularly around the abdomen, increases pressure on the stomach, which can force stomach acid up into the *esophagus*, leading to heartburn. By aiding in weight loss and the reduction of abdominal fat, regular physical activity can decrease the likelihood of acid reflux episodes. Aerobic exercises such as walking, jogging, swimming, or cycling are particularly effective for burning calories and promoting a healthy weight, thereby reducing the risk of heartburn.

**Stress Reduction -** Stress is a known trigger for heartburn, as it can increase stomach acid production and lead to behaviors that exacerbate acid reflux, such as overeating or consuming trigger foods. Exercise is a powerful stress reliever, releasing *endorphins*, the body's natural painkillers and mood elevators. Activities like yoga and Pilates, in addition to aerobic exercises, can significantly lower stress levels, thus indirectly preventing heartburn by reducing one of its key triggers.

**Strengthening the Digestive System** - Regular exercise can improve gastrointestinal (GI) health in several ways. It enhances blood flow to the digestive tract, which can help the stomach and intestines function more efficiently, reducing the likelihood of conditions such as constipation and bloating, which can increase the risk of heartburn. Furthermore, certain exercises can strengthen the abdominal muscles, supporting the GI tract and improving posture, which in turn can help prevent the reflux of stomach acid.

## Exercise Considerations

While exercise can prevent heartburn, it's important to choose the right types and timing of activities. High-impact exercises or those involving bending over can increase abdominal pressure and potentially worsen heartburn immediately after eating. It's advisable to wait at least two hours after a meal before engaging in vigorous exercise and to stay hydrated with water, avoiding caffeinated beverages that can increase stomach acidity.

In conclusion, regular exercise plays a crucial role in preventing heartburn through weight management, stress reduction, and the strengthening of the digestive system. Incorporating a balanced mix of aerobic and stress-reducing exercises into one's routine can offer a natural and effective way to manage heartburn symptoms. However, it's important to tailor exercise choices to individual health status and to consult with healthcare professionals when necessary, ensuring that physical activity contributes positively to overall digestive health and well-being.

## **Adequate Sleep:** Adequate Sleep plays a crucial role in maintaining overall health and can be particularly effective in preventing heartburn, a common symptom of acid reflux. Poor sleep patterns and sleep deprivation have been linked to an increase in stress and inflammation in the body, which can exacerbate gastrointestinal issues, including heartburn. When the body is well-rested, it's better equipped to manage stress and regulate the hormones that influence digestion and stomach acid production.

Furthermore, a lack of sleep can lead to unhealthy eating habits, such as late-night snacking or choosing foods that trigger heartburn. These behaviors increase the likelihood of experiencing acid reflux. By ensuring adequate sleep, individuals are more likely to make healthier eating choices and avoid late meals, reducing the risk of heartburn.

Prioritizing adequate sleep contributes to stress reduction, healthier lifestyle choices, and improved digestive health, all of which are beneficial in preventing heartburn. Ensuring a regular sleep schedule and creating a conducive sleep environment are simple yet effective strategies to reduce the risk of heartburn and enhance overall well-being.

# Effective Time Management:

Effective Time Management plays a surprisingly significant role in preventing heartburn as well, primarily by reducing stress and promoting healthier eating habits. Stress can often result from feeling overwhelmed by tasks and deadlines. By efficiently managing time, individuals can significantly lower their stress levels, thereby reducing the likelihood of stress-induced acid reflux.

Moreover, good time management allows for more thoughtful meal planning and prevents rushed eating or reliance on fast food, which are common when time feels scarce. Eating in a relaxed state, chewing food thoroughly, and allowing sufficient time between eating and physical activity or sleep can greatly minimize the risk of heartburn. It encourages regular, smaller meals rather than large, heavy meals that can put extra pressure on the stomach, leading to acid reflux. In essence, by adopting effective time management strategies, individuals can create a more balanced lifestyle, reducing stress and promoting healthier eating patterns, which in turn can help prevent the occurrence of heartburn.

**<u>Social Support:</u>** Social support plays a pivotal role in managing and preventing heartburn, primarily through its impact on stress reduction and emotional well-being. Interacting with friends, family, and support groups can provide emotional comfort, reduce feelings of isolation, and offer practical advice for managing stress, which is a known trigger for acid reflux and heartburn. When individuals feel supported, they are more likely to engage in positive health behaviors and less likely to resort to stress-related eating habits that can exacerbate heartburn, such as consuming spicy, fatty, or acidic foods.

Also something to think about, social interactions can encourage adherence to treatment plans and lifestyle modifications recommended for managing heartburn. Sharing experiences and coping strategies with others who have similar conditions can lead to the discovery of effective heartburn management techniques and provide a sense of community and understanding. Additionally, laughter and positive social engagements have been shown to boost mood and reduce stress, further mitigating the risk of heartburn.

In summary, leveraging social support can for many contribute to the prevention of heartburn by fostering stress resilience, promoting healthy behaviors, and providing a platform for emotional and practical support. This underscores the importance of maintaining strong social connections as part of a comprehensive approach to managing heartburn and enhancing overall well-being.

# Hobbies and Leisure Activities:

Hobbies and leisure activities are vital for stress management, directly impacting the prevention of heartburn. These activities, ranging from creative arts to outdoor adventures, serve as effective stress relievers, reducing the body's stress response that often exacerbates acid reflux symptoms. Engaging in enjoyable pursuits facilitates relaxation, lowers the production of stress hormones that can increase stomach acid, and promotes a positive mood.

This psychological and physiological relaxation can encourage healthier lifestyle choices that contribute to better digestive health. Thus, incorporating leisure activities into daily life can be a simple yet powerful strategy to combat heartburn.

---

Incorporating these many stress reduction techniques into your daily routine can not only help manage heartburn but also improve overall health and quality of life. It's important to note that while stress reduction can aid in managing heartburn, it should complement other treatments and lifestyle adjustments recommended by healthcare professionals for comprehensive management of acid reflux.

# Chiropractic Care:

*Chiropractic care*, often associated with the treatment of back pain and musculoskeletal issues, can also offer benefits for individuals suffering from heartburn or *(GERD)*. This approach is rooted in the principle that proper alignment of the body's musculoskeletal structure, particularly the spine, can enable the body to heal itself without the need for surgery or medication. By addressing the structural causes of heartburn, chiropractic treatments can provide a non-invasive, holistic option for managing and potentially preventing this condition.

## Chiropractic Approach to Heartburn

Chiropractors focus on correcting spinal misalignments *(subluxations)* that can interfere with the nervous system's regulation of bodily functions, including digestion. By restoring proper alignment, chiropractic care can improve nerve function, which in turn may enhance the digestive process and prevent the relaxation of the *lower esophageal sphincter (LES)* that typically allows acid to reflux into the *esophagus*.

## Techniques and Benefits

1. **Spinal Adjustments:** The core of chiropractic care, spinal adjustments, can relieve pressure on nerves that control digestive functions. This can lead to improved signaling between the brain and

digestive system, enhancing LES function and preventing heartburn.

2. **Soft Tissue Therapy:** Chiropractors may use soft tissue techniques to relieve tension in the abdominal and diaphragmatic muscles. Reducing this tension can improve diaphragm function, which is crucial for maintaining the correct position of stomach contents and preventing reflux.

3. **Postural Correction:** Poor posture can exacerbate heartburn by increasing abdominal pressure and encouraging acid reflux. Chiropractic care often includes postural advice and exercises that strengthen the core and improve posture, thereby reducing the risk of heartburn.

4. **Lifestyle and Dietary Advice:** Chiropractors may provide holistic care that includes lifestyle and dietary recommendations to support digestive health. This might involve advice on foods to avoid, eating habits to adopt, and exercises that can strengthen the body's core and reduce stress.

## Clinical Evidence and Considerations

While research on chiropractic care for heartburn is still evolving, anecdotal evidence and preliminary studies suggest it can be an effective complementary treatment.

Patients with heartburn who have undergone chiropractic adjustments often report improvements in their symptoms, attributed to the enhanced nervous system function and reduced mechanical stress on the digestive tract.

However, it's important to note that chiropractic care should be considered part of a comprehensive approach to managing heartburn, which may also include dietary changes, medication, and other lifestyle adjustments. Individuals considering chiropractic treatment for heartburn should consult with a healthcare professional to ensure it's an appropriate option for their specific condition.

## Potential Risks and Limitations

As with any treatment, chiropractic care comes with potential risks and limitations. It's essential for individuals to seek care from licensed and experienced chiropractors. While adverse effects are rare, they can occur, particularly if treatments are not performed correctly.

## To Summarize

Chiropractic care offers a unique, holistic approach to preventing and managing heartburn. Through spinal adjustments, soft tissue therapy, postural correction, and comprehensive lifestyle advice, chiropractors can address some of the root causes of acid reflux. By improving spinal alignment, enhancing nervous system function, and reducing mechanical stress on the digestive system, chiropractic treatments may help alleviate heartburn symptoms and improve overall digestive health.

As the medical community continues to explore the benefits of chiropractic care for a range of conditions, including heartburn, it becomes increasingly clear that this approach can be a valuable component of a holistic health strategy. For those seeking alternative or complementary treatments to traditional heartburn medications, chiropractic care presents an option worth considering, offering the potential for relief through natural, body-centered healing practices.

# NINE
## Quick at Home Treatments

Here are some lesser-known home remedies for heartburn, utilizing items you likely already have available at home. These include solutions for quick relief and daily preventive strategies.

## **Baking Soda**

Baking soda, or **sodium bicarbonate**, is a common household item that can offer quick relief from heartburn. Baking soda's effectiveness lies in its basicity; it acts as a natural *antacid* by neutralizing stomach acid, thereby providing temporary relief from the discomfort associated with heartburn.

The process is simple: when baking soda is dissolved in water, it reacts with the *hydrochloric acid* in the stomach to form salt, water, and carbon dioxide. This reaction increases the pH level of the stomach contents, making it less acidic and alleviating the burning sensation typically felt during heartburn episodes.

***How to use:*** Dissolve half a teaspoon of it in a glass of water and drink it slowly. It's important to measure the baking soda carefully and not to overuse this remedy, as consuming large amounts can cause serious *electrolyte* and acid/base imbalances. Also, because the reaction produces carbon dioxide gas, it may lead to belching or bloating.

While baking soda can provide quick relief, it's a temporary solution and not a cure for underlying digestive issues. It's also not recommended for frequent use or as a long-term solution for heartburn. Individuals with high blood pressure or on a sodium-restricted diet should avoid using baking soda due to its high sodium content. Always consult with a healthcare professional before trying new remedies, especially if you experience heartburn regularly.

## <u>Oatmeal</u>

Oatmeal is a beneficial food for those suffering from heartburn, thanks to its ability to absorb excess stomach acid and its high fiber content, which aids in digestion. As a whole grain, oatmeal helps maintain a healthy digestive tract, ensuring smoother passage of food through the stomach and reducing the risk of acid reflux, which of course is the primary cause of heartburn. Its soothing properties and ability to provide a protective coating for the lining of the *esophagus* and stomach further contribute to its effectiveness in managing heartburn symptoms.

***How to use***: Start your day with a bowl of plain, cooked oatmeal. Avoid adding ingredients that are known triggers for heartburn, such as high-fat dairy products, citrus fruits, or chocolate. Instead, you can sweeten your oatmeal with a bit of honey or top it with alkaline fruits like bananas to enhance its beneficial effects. Eating oatmeal regularly can not only help manage heartburn but also contribute to overall digestive health.

## **Mustard**

Despite being based more on personal testimony than scientific proof *(anecdotal)*, mustard is touted by many as a handy remedy for heartburn. This yellow condiment is believed to neutralize stomach acid thanks to its vinegar content and minerals, potentially offering quick relief from the burn.

***How to use:*** Swallow a teaspoon of plain yellow mustard when heartburn strikes. It's a simple, if unconventional, method that some swear by for instant alleviation of heartburn symptoms. Keep in mind, though, results can vary, and it's always wise to approach such anecdotal remedies with a bit of caution.

## **Water**

Yes WATER can be a surprisingly effective remedy for heartburn by diluting stomach acid and helping to flush it from the *esophagus*, providing immediate relief from the burning sensation. Simply drinking a full glass of water when you start feeling the symptoms of heartburn can help minimize the discomfort. It's a straightforward and natural approach that aids in digestion and can prevent the accumulation of acid. For best results, drink water throughout the day to maintain hydration and support digestive health.

## Almonds

Almonds are often cited as a natural remedy for heartburn, offering both immediate relief and potential long-term benefits for digestive health. This nutrient-rich nut contains natural oils that can soothe the stomach and neutralize stomach acid, reducing the discomfort associated with heartburn. The theory behind almonds' effectiveness lies in their ability to balance the body's pH levels, making the stomach environment less acidic and thereby minimizing the risk of acid reflux.

To utilize almonds for heartburn relief, consuming a small handful of raw or roasted almonds after meals or when heartburn symptoms arise is recommended. The act of chewing almonds thoroughly increases saliva production, which can help neutralize stomach acid. Additionally, almonds are a good source of fiber, which aids in digestion and promotes a healthy gastrointestinal tract, further preventing episodes of heartburn.

It's important to note that while many people find almonds to be a helpful remedy for heartburn, individual responses can vary. For some, especially those with nut allergies or sensitivities, almonds may not be a suitable option. As with any dietary approach to managing heartburn, moderation is key, and integrating almonds as part of a balanced diet can contribute to overall digestive wellness and symptom management.

## Bananas

Bananas are a gentle, natural antacid, providing relief from heartburn by coating the stomach lining and protecting it from acid. Their high potassium content helps to neutralize stomach acid, reducing discomfort. Moreover, bananas are rich in *pectin*, a soluble fiber that aids digestion and movement of food through the digestive tract more smoothly, preventing acid reflux episodes.

For heartburn relief, eating a ripe banana can offer immediate soothing effects. Ripe bananas are preferable as they are less acidic and more alkaline, making them more effective in countering heartburn. Incorporating bananas into your daily diet can also serve as a preventive measure against heartburn, thanks to their overall contribution to improved digestive health. Simple and convenient, bananas are an excellent remedy for those seeking a natural approach to managing heartburn.

# TEN
## Out-of-the-Box Concepts

Thus far, we've looked into numerous methods to ease heartburn. While some suggestions offer instant relief and can be quickly adopted, others necessitate careful planning and consideration. A few strategies even call for in-depth research or consultations with holistic health professionals.

The goal is to present a broad array of effective solutions, ensuring that you find at least one or many more that prove beneficial. In this final segment before discussing medical treatments, we'll introduce several additional unconventional strategies that have shown promise for many.

## **Singing or Humming**

Singing or humming might seem unconventional, but these activities can indirectly help alleviate heartburn by promoting relaxation and reducing stress, a known trigger for acid reflux. The act of singing or humming encourages deep breathing, which can improve diaphragm movement and support better digestion.

Additionally, these vocal activities can increase saliva production, which helps neutralize stomach acid. To try this method, simply hum your favorite tune or sing softly to yourself, especially after meals or when feeling stressed. This natural, soothing practice not only reduces stress levels but may also offer a unique way to manage heartburn symptoms through improved respiratory and digestive function.

# Laughter Yoga

*Laughter Yoga* (yes this is a real thing), combines laughter exercises with yogic breathing (**Pranayama**), offering a unique approach to alleviating heartburn. Laughing intensely can stimulate digestion and enhance oxygen intake, reducing stress and potentially lowering the acidity in the stomach.

To practice Laughter Yoga, join a group or find online sessions where guided laughter exercises encourage genuine and contagious laughter. Regular participation can promote relaxation, improve digestion, and as a result, help manage heartburn symptoms. This enjoyable and communal activity underscores laughter's role in holistic well-being, including digestive health.

# Aromatherapy

*Aromatherapy*, the practice of using essential oils for therapeutic benefits, can be a supportive measure in managing heartburn, primarily through stress reduction and promoting relaxation. Stress is a significant trigger for acid reflux, as it can lead to an increase in stomach acid production and tension in the digestive tract. By alleviating stress, aromatherapy may indirectly help prevent heartburn episodes.

Essential oils such as lavender, ginger, lemon, and peppermint are particularly noted for their soothing properties on the digestive system. Lavender oil is renowned for its ability to promote relaxation and reduce anxiety. Ginger oil can aid digestion and soothe stomach discomfort. Lemon oil has natural detoxifying properties and can help balance stomach acid levels. Peppermint oil, while beneficial for some, should be used with caution as it can exacerbate heartburn in certain individuals.

To use aromatherapy for heartburn relief, you can diffuse the essential oils in your living space, apply diluted oils topically to your abdomen or chest (after ensuring no allergic reactions), or inhale the aroma directly from the bottle or a handkerchief. It's important to use high-quality, pure essential oils and dilute them appropriately with a carrier oil if applied topically to avoid skin irritation.

While aromatherapy can provide symptomatic relief and contribute to a holistic approach to managing heartburn, it should not replace treatments recommended by healthcare professionals. It's best used as a complementary therapy alongside dietary changes, lifestyle modifications, and any prescribed medications for a comprehensive management plan.

## Posture Training

Posture training plays a crucial role in managing heartburn by aligning the body in a way that minimizes acid reflux. Poor posture, especially while sitting or bending over, can compress the stomach and force acid into the *esophagus*, leading to heartburn. By improving posture, you can reduce this pressure and prevent reflux.

To incorporate posture training for heartburn relief, focus on maintaining a straight back with shoulders back and down, whether sitting or standing. Use ergonomic chairs that support spinal alignment and take frequent breaks to stretch if you spend long hours at a desk. Additionally, avoid slouching or lying down immediately after eating. Instead, walk or stand to encourage digestion.

Practicing exercises that strengthen the core muscles, such as *Pilates* or *Yoga*, can also support better posture. These activities not only enhance abdominal strength but also promote awareness of body alignment, further aiding in the prevention of heartburn.

## Chewing Gum with Bicarbonate

Chewing gum with *bicarbonate* (baking soda) can be an effective way to alleviate heartburn. This simple activity stimulates saliva production, which helps neutralize stomach acid and wash it back down into the stomach, providing relief from the burning sensation. The *bicarbonate* in the gum enhances this neutralizing effect. For best results, chew a piece of gum with bicarbonate for about 30 minutes after meals to prevent heartburn symptoms. This method is easy, convenient, and can be particularly helpful in managing acid reflux after eating.

## Acupressure Wristbands

*Acupressure wristbands*, commonly used to alleviate motion sickness and nausea, can also offer relief from heartburn symptoms through the principles of acupressure. These wristbands apply continuous pressure to specific points on the wrist, particularly the *Nei-Kuan (P6) point*, which is believed to regulate the flow of energy and help balance the body's digestive functions.

The *Nei-Kuan point* is located three finger widths below the wrist on the inner forearm in between the two tendons. By stimulating this point, acupressure wristbands can help soothe the stomach and reduce the incidence of acid reflux, which in turn alleviates heartburn. This method is non-invasive and serves as a natural remedy to manage digestive discomfort.

To use acupressure wristbands for heartburn, place the band on each wrist with the pressure button facing downward, directly over the Nei-Kuan point. Wear the bands throughout the day or specifically after meals when heartburn is more likely to occur. While the effectiveness of acupressure wristbands can vary from person to person, many find them a convenient and drug-free option for managing heartburn. They are especially useful for pregnant women or others seeking an alternative to medication. However, it's always wise to consult with a healthcare provider before trying new remedies for heartburn.

## **Virtual Reality (VR)**

*Virtual Reality (VR)* relaxation is an innovative approach to managing heartburn by reducing stress and anxiety, which are significant triggers for acid reflux. Immersive VR environments transport users to calming landscapes or scenarios, facilitating deep relaxation and distraction from discomfort. This stress relief can potentially decrease stomach acid production, mitigating heartburn symptoms.

To use VR for relaxation, wear a VR headset and select a relaxation or meditation program designed to promote calmness. Engage in these sessions regularly or during episodes of heartburn for maximum benefit. This technology offers a novel, immersive way to manage stress and its physical manifestations, including heartburn, through virtual escapism.

# Cold Showers

Cold showers can offer an unexpected benefit for heartburn sufferers by enhancing circulation and stimulating the *vagus nerve*, which plays a role in managing digestion and reducing stress levels. The shock of cold water on the body can also divert attention from heartburn discomfort, providing a form of temporary relief.

To use this method, start with a lukewarm shower and gradually decrease the water temperature to cold. Aim to stay under the cold water for a few minutes, focusing on deep, controlled breathing to maximize the calming effect on the digestive system. Regular cold showers may not only help in managing heartburn symptoms but also improve overall vitality and stress resilience, contributing to better digestive health.

# Left Side Sleeping

Sleeping on the left side is a simple yet effective method for alleviating heartburn symptoms. This position takes advantage of the stomach's natural anatomy, positioning it in a way that makes acid less likely to escape into the *esophagus*. The benefit comes from gravity's role in aiding digestion and preventing the backflow of stomach contents.

To adopt left-side sleeping, use a supportive pillow to ensure comfort and maintain alignment throughout the night. Starting this habit may require some adjustment, but consistently sleeping on your left side can significantly reduce the frequency and intensity of heartburn episodes, promoting a more restful and comfortable sleep.

# Foot Massage

Foot massage, surprisingly, can be an indirect yet effective approach to alleviating heartburn symptoms, rooted in the principles of *Reflexology*. This technique posits that points on the feet are connected to various organs and systems throughout the body, including the digestive system. By massaging specific points on the feet that correspond to the stomach and *esophagus*, it's believed that foot massage can help soothe digestive issues and reduce heartburn.

To utilize foot massage for heartburn relief, focus on the arches of your feet, which are linked to the digestive organs. Applying gentle pressure and circular motions in these areas can stimulate digestion and potentially ease the discomfort associated with acid reflux. Additionally, the overall relaxation effect of a foot massage can lower stress levels, a known trigger for heartburn.

Incorporating foot massage into your routine can be as simple as dedicating a few minutes each day to self-massage or enlisting the help of a partner. For those interested in a more targeted approach, consulting with a *reflexologist* who can accurately identify and apply pressure to the specific reflex points associated with heartburn may provide more pronounced relief. Beyond its potential digestive benefits, foot massage offers a holistic way to relax and promote overall well-being.

# In Conclusion

Exploring every non-medical, innovative method to alleviate heartburn is a commendable strategy, offering a broad spectrum of potential solutions without immediately resorting to medication.

Such approaches, ranging from dietary adjustments and lifestyle changes to stress-reduction techniques and natural remedies, can provide significant relief with minimal risk of side effects. They empower individuals to take control of their health through holistic means, encouraging a deeper understanding of their bodies and how various factors influence digestive health.

By considering these alternative strategies, you not only stand to reduce heartburn symptoms but also improve overall well-being. It's a proactive approach that fosters a healthier, more balanced lifestyle, making it a valuable consideration for anyone struggling with heartburn.

# MEDICAL REMEDIES

## <u>Introduction</u>

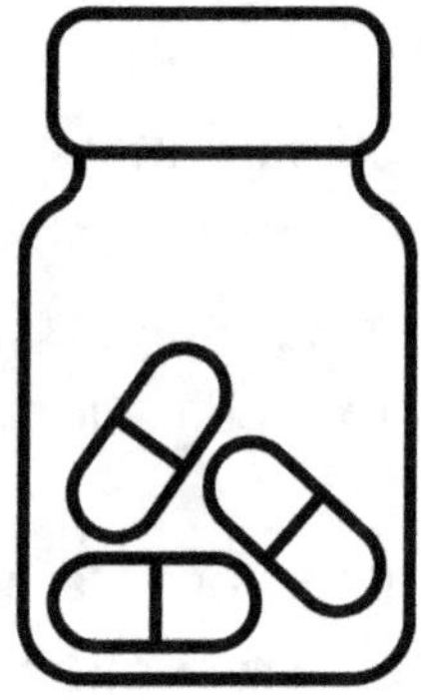

Upon concluding this section, the aim is for you to gain fresh insights and abilities in navigating the pharmacy's massive array of heartburn and acid reflux remedies. The multitude of brands and formulations available will no longer seem like a perplexing puzzle.

Instead, you'll have the knowledge to discern the active ingredients in each product, understand the type of medication they represent, and make an informed decision about which one is likely to be most effective for your needs. I recommend taking this book along as a reference when you go to any pharmacy.

If you're currently utilizing a heartburn/GERD treatment, this section will enhance your understanding of what you're taking, the compounds it uses, and whether it's the right choice for you.

Additionally, you'll gain knowledge about generic versus brand-name medications, understanding any quality differences and the reasons behind the significant price disparities. Grasping these points alone, makes this book an exceptional resource.

---

*An effective strategy to utilize this portion of the book is to explore and study the ingredients in your own medicines. Additionally, when in any store pharmacy section you can identify the ingredients or compounds used in a wide variety of medicines, both generic and name brand.*

*Simply find the medical compound's name in the back of this book's **'Glossary of Terms'** (e.g., Cimetidine - page 218), then go directly to the provided page. This approach will quickly take you to the information on the type of medication you're looking at, how that medication functions, and its advantages and disadvantages.*

---

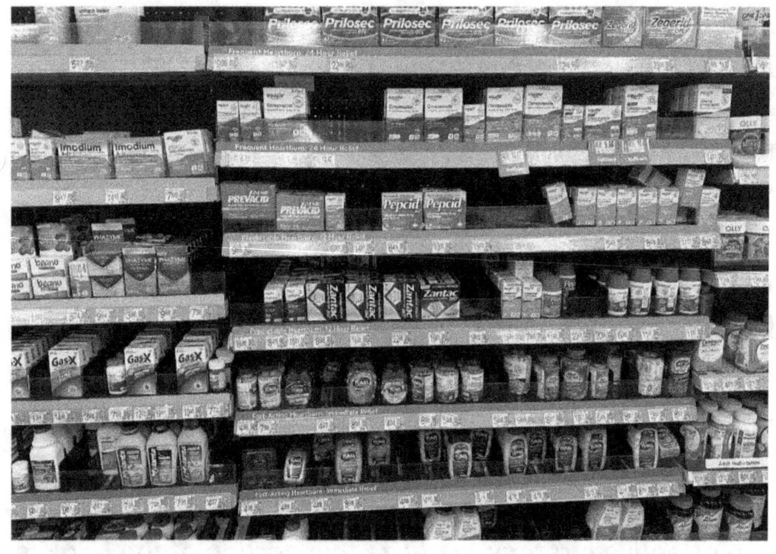

"The vast selection of medicines, while a testament to advancements in healthcare, often leaves us feeling lost amid a sea of choices"

Deciding on the right medication becomes a daunting task, compounded by the massive numbers of brands, generics, dosages, and forms available. It's a scenario that reflects our times—where an abundance of options doesn't necessarily translate to clarity, but rather to a complex puzzle that each of us is tasked with solving.

# ELEVEN
## Types of Medications

In the following sections we will explore:

**1. The 6 primary types of medications, and their *"Mechanism of Action"***

☐ Antacids
☐ H2 Blockers
☐ Proton Pump Inhibitors (PPIs)
☐ Prokinetics
☐ Alginates
☐ Coating Agents

**2. Prominent brand names and the active ingredients they use.**

**3. A component analysis with pros and cons of each of those ingredients.**

# Antacids
## Tums, Rolaids, Mylanta, Alka-Seltzer-Heartburn Relief, Gaviscon

The *mechanism of action* of antacids is relatively simple. When they are ingested, they quickly dissolve in the stomach and react with *gastric acid* to increase the *pH level* of the stomach contents. This reduction in acidity can provide rapid relief from the discomfort associated with excess stomach acid.

They are available over the counter and are commonly used.

The main active ingredients in antacids include: *magnesium hydroxide, aluminum hydroxide, calcium carbonate*, and *sodium bicarbonate*. Each of these compounds works by reacting with stomach acid (*hydrochloric acid*) to form water and other neutral compounds, thereby reducing the acidity in the stomach.

However, because antacids work by neutralizing acid after it is already in the stomach, they do not prevent acid production. Therefore, their effect is temporary, and they may need to be taken frequently to manage symptoms.

Antacids can also affect the absorption of certain medications and nutrients, making it important to manage the timing of their intake. They are generally safe for most people when used as directed, but long-term reliance on antacids for symptom management should be discussed with a healthcare provider to explore more effective and sustainable treatment options for acid-related disorders.

~~~~~~~~~~~~~~~~~~~~~~~~~~~~~~~~~~

While antacids are effective for occasional use, understanding their benefits and drawbacks is important for safe and optimal relief.

~~~~~~~~~~~~~~~~~~~~~~~~~~~~~~~~~~

# Antacid Medicines

Below are a few recognized and commonly available antacid brands in various regions. Keep in mind that availability may vary by location, and new products may come onto the market while others may be discontinued.

**Tums:** *Tums* primarily contain *calcium carbonate* as its active ingredient. It may also contain other ingredients such as binders, flavors, and colorings to enhance the product's taste and appearance, but the main medicinal component is calcium carbonate.

**Rolaids:** *Rolaids* typically contain two active ingredients: *Calcium Carbonate* and *Magnesium Hydroxide*. These compounds work together as antacids to neutralize stomach acid. *Calcium carbonate* acts by neutralizing excess stomach acid, while *magnesium hydroxide* can induce a laxative effect, which can help counteract any potential constipation caused by calcium carbonate. Together, they offer effective relief from discomfort caused by acid-related issues.

**Mylanta:** The active ingredients typically found in *Mylanta* include: *Aluminum Hydroxide*, *Magnesium Hydroxide*, and *Simethicone*. These ingredients work together to provide relief from discomfort caused by excess stomach acid and gas, making Mylanta a comprehensive treatment for multiple symptoms associated with heartburn and acid reflux. The combination of *aluminum hydroxide* and *magnesium hydroxide* offers a balanced antacid effect, while *simethicone* helps manage gas-related symptoms.

## Alka-Seltzer - Heartburn Relief:

*Alka-Seltzer-Heartburn Relief* products are formulated specifically to address heartburn and acid indigestion. Unlike the classic Alka-Seltzer, which contains aspirin, sodium bicarbonate, and citric acid, Alka-Seltzer Heartburn Relief formulations typically do not contain aspirin. Instead, they focus on neutralizing stomach acid quickly. The specific compounds used in Alka-Seltzer Heartburn Relief products may vary, but common active ingredients may include : *Sodium Bicarbonate* and *Calcium Carbonate*: Some versions of Alka-Seltzer Heartburn Relief might also include other ingredients aimed at addressing additional symptoms or providing faster relief. It's important to read the label of the specific product you're using to understand its active ingredients and intended use.

## Gaviscon: The active ingredients in *Gaviscon* vary

slightly depending on the formulation and the country in which it is sold, but generally, Gaviscon products may contain: *Aluminum Hydroxide*, *Magnesium Carbonate* and *Sodium Alginate*. These ingredients work together to provide relief from the symptoms of acid reflux and heartburn by neutralizing stomach acid and forming a protective barrier to prevent acid from re-entering the *esophagus*. Gaviscon is available in various forms, including tablets and liquid. Always refer to the specific product label for the most accurate information on active ingredients.

# Antacids
## Compounds Used – Pros & Cons

Calcium Carbonate, Magnesium Hydroxide, Aluminum Hydroxide, Sodium Bicarbonate, Simethicone

**Calcium Carbonate:** *Calcium carbonate* is a widely prevalent compound found naturally in rocks, pearls, and the shells of marine organisms. Its chemical formula is $CaCO_3$, embodying a combination of calcium, carbon, and oxygen. This compound is the principal component of limestone, chalk, and marble, three of the most common forms of *calcium carbonate* found in nature. Due to its vast availability and versatile properties, calcium carbonate has a broad range of applications both industrially and medically.

In the medical field, calcium carbonate is extensively used as a calcium supplement and antacid. As a supplement, it helps prevent and treat calcium deficiencies and conditions related to low bone density, such as *osteoporosis*. Its antacid properties offer quick relief from symptoms of heartburn, acid indigestion, and upset stomach by neutralizing stomach acid.

Furthermore, calcium carbonate is favored for its high calcium content and cost-effectiveness, making it a popular choice among calcium supplements. However, its effectiveness as a calcium source is dependent on stomach acid for absorption, making it less suitable for individuals with reduced stomach acid levels.

Interestingly, besides its medical uses, calcium carbonate is also a critical ingredient in the manufacture of cement and lime, and as a filler and coating agent in the production of paper, plastics, and paint, showcasing its versatility across various industries.

## Pros

1. **Effective Antacid:** It quickly neutralizes stomach acid, providing relief from heartburn, acid indigestion, and an upset stomach.

2. **Calcium Supplementation:** As a source of calcium, it helps in the prevention and treatment of *osteoporosis* by supporting bone health and maintenance.

3. **Cost-Effective:** Compared to other calcium supplements, calcium carbonate is relatively inexpensive and widely available.

4. **Versatile Forms:** Available in various forms (tablets, capsules, chewables, liquids), making it accessible for different age groups and preferences.

# <u>Cons</u>

1. **Absorption Issues:** *Calcium carbonate* requires stomach acid for best absorption, so it may be less effective when taken on an empty stomach or for individuals with low stomach acid.

2. **Gastrointestinal Side Effects:** Can cause gas, bloating, and constipation in some individuals, especially when taken in high doses.

3. **Risk of Overuse:** Excessive consumption can lead to *hypercalcemia* (high calcium levels in the blood), which can affect kidney function and lead to kidney stones.

4. **Interactions:** It can interfere with the absorption of other medications, such as bisphosphonates (used to treat osteoporosis) and some antibiotics, reducing their effectiveness.

In medical use, the choice to use *calcium carbonate* should consider these pros and cons, balancing its benefits against potential side effects or interactions with other medications. It's important for individuals to consult healthcare professionals before starting any new supplement, especially if they have underlying health conditions or are taking other medications.

# Magnesium Hydroxide: *Magnesium hydroxide* is an inorganic compound commonly used as an antacid and a **laxative**, recognized for its ability to neutralize stomach acid and relieve symptoms of indigestion, heartburn, and sour stomach. It works by reacting with *hydrochloric acid* in the stomach to form **magnesium chloride** and water, thereby reducing acidity and providing symptomatic relief from discomfort caused by excess stomach acid.

As a laxative, *magnesium hydroxide* operates by drawing water into the intestines, which helps to soften the stool and promotes intestinal movements, aiding in the relief of occasional constipation.

Available over the counter in various forms, including liquid suspensions and tablets, magnesium hydroxide is known for its quick onset of action and safety profile when used as directed. However, it's essential for users to adhere to recommended dosages to avoid potential side effects such as diarrhea or *electrolyte imbalances*. Long-term use or overuse should be avoided unless supervised by a healthcare provider, as it may lead to dependency for bowel function or affect the balance of minerals in the body.

# **<u>Pros</u>**

1. **Effective Antacid:** *Magnesium hydroxide* quickly neutralizes stomach acid, providing relief from indigestion, heartburn, and acid reflux. This can improve quality of life for those suffering from these conditions.

2. **Gentle Laxative:** As a laxative, it works by drawing water into the intestines, which helps soften the stool and promotes bowel movements. This mechanism is gentle and considered safe for occasional use.

3. **Minimal Systemic Absorption:** It has minimal systemic absorption, which makes it a safer option compared to other medications that are absorbed into the bloodstream and may have widespread effects.

4. **Availability:** It is readily available over the counter in various forms, making it easily accessible for those in need of quick relief.

5. **Safe for Kidneys:** In patients with normal kidney function, it can be safer than other antacids that contain aluminum or calcium, which can cause problems in individuals with renal issues.

# <u>Cons</u>

1. **Hypermagnesemia Risk:** In patients with renal impairment, there's a risk of *hypermagnesemia* (high magnesium levels in the blood) due to decreased ability to excrete magnesium, which can lead to serious side effects.

2. **Diarrhea:** Overuse as a laxative can lead to diarrhea, which may result in dehydration and electrolyte imbalances if not properly managed.

3. **Interactions with Medications:** Magnesium hydroxide can interfere with the absorption of certain medications, including some antibiotics and bisphosphonates, reducing their effectiveness.

4. **Dependency:** With prolonged use as a laxative, there's a risk of becoming dependent on it for bowel movements, potentially leading to a cycle where natural bowel function is diminished.

5. **Limited Long-Term Use:** Due to potential side effects and interactions, magnesium hydroxide is not recommended for long-term use without medical supervision.

In summary, magnesium hydroxide offers significant benefits for treating acid-related disorders and constipation with minimal side effects when used appropriately. However, its cons highlight the importance of careful and informed use, especially in individuals with underlying health conditions or those taking other medications.

## Aluminum Hydroxide: *Aluminum hydroxide* is an antacid medication commonly used to treat symptoms of excess stomach acid, such as heartburn, acid indigestion, and upset stomach. It works by neutralizing stomach acid, thereby providing relief from discomfort. Beyond its antacid properties, *aluminum hydroxide* is also used to reduce **phosphate levels** in people with certain kidney conditions, helping to prevent the formation of kidney stones by binding phosphate in the intestines.

Available in various forms, including tablets, capsules, and liquid suspensions, aluminum hydroxide is accessible and easy to use. However, it's important for users to follow dosing instructions carefully to avoid side effects such as constipation, which is a common issue with aluminum-containing antacids. In some cases, long-term use can lead to aluminum accumulation, particularly in individuals with kidney problems, leading to potential health risks. Therefore, while aluminum hydroxide is effective for temporary relief of stomach acid-related symptoms, it should be used judiciously and under the guidance of a healthcare professional, especially for individuals with pre-existing health conditions.

*Aluminum hydroxide* is commonly used in medicine as an antacid and ***phosphate binder***, offering relief from symptoms of increased stomach acidity such as heartburn, upset stomach, and indigestion. It also helps reduce phosphate levels in people with certain kidney conditions.

## **Pros**

1. **Effective Antacid:** *Aluminum hydroxide* effectively neutralizes stomach acid, providing quick relief from acid-related symptoms.

2. **Phosphate Binder:** It is beneficial for patients with chronic kidney disease by reducing phosphate absorption in the intestines, thus helping manage *serum phosphate levels*.

3. **Safety Profile:** Generally considered safe for short-term use in appropriate doses, with minimal systemic absorption.

4. **Versatile Use:** Available in various forms, such as tablets, capsules, and liquid, making it accessible for different patient needs and preferences.

# Cons

1. **Constipation:** One of the most common side effects is constipation, which can be uncomfortable and require management with diet or medication.

2. **Potential for Aluminum Toxicity:** With long-term use, especially in patients with renal impairment, there's a risk of aluminum accumulation leading to toxicity, affecting the central nervous system and bones.

3. **Drug Interactions:** *Aluminum hydroxide* can interfere with the absorption of several medications, including antibiotics and heart medications, potentially reducing their effectiveness.

4. **Nutrient Absorption:** It may also interfere with the absorption of certain nutrients, such as iron, leading to deficiencies if used over a long period.

While *aluminum hydroxide* can be an effective treatment for managing symptoms of excess stomach acid and controlling phosphate levels in kidney patients, its use should be carefully considered against potential side effects and interactions. It's important for patients to follow medical advice to minimize risks.

# Sodium Bicarbonate: *Sodium*

*Bicarbonate* commonly known as baking soda, is a versatile compound with a wide range of uses, including medical applications. Chemically, it is represented as $NaHCO_3$ and is a white, crystalline powder that is slightly alkaline in taste. In the medical field, *sodium bicarbonate* is primarily used as an antacid to treat conditions like heartburn, acid indigestion, and upset stomach by neutralizing stomach acid, providing quick relief from discomfort.

Beyond its antacid properties, *sodium bicarbonate* is also utilized in emergency medicine as an intravenous infusion to correct ***acidosis*** in patients with severe ***metabolic acidosis***, a condition where the body produces excessive acid or the kidneys are not removing enough acid from the body.

Additionally, it serves a role in the treatment of certain drug intoxications, including ***Tricyclic Antidepressant Overdose***, by helping to normalize the body's pH balance. Despite its benefits, careful administration is necessary to avoid side effects, such as metabolic alkalosis, especially in patients with underlying health conditions.

*Sodium bicarbonate*, widely known as baking soda, is used medically for its antacid properties and ability to manage acid-base imbalances. Here are the pros and cons of its medical use:

# Pros

1. **Rapid Acid Neutralization:** *Sodium bicarbonate* effectively neutralizes stomach acid, providing quick relief from conditions like heartburn, acid indigestion, and upset stomach.

2. **Treatment of Acidosis:** It is used in emergency medicine to correct *metabolic acidosis*, a condition where the body has too much acid, helping to restore the body's pH balance.

3. **Versatile Medical Uses:** Beyond treating acid-related conditions, it's used in the management of certain drug overdoses and poisoning by helping to increase the pH of urine, which facilitates the excretion of certain substances.

4. **Availability:** It is readily available, inexpensive, and can be administered orally or intravenously, making it accessible for a variety of medical situations.

# Cons

1. **Electrolyte Imbalance:** With excessive use, *sodium bicarbonate* can lead to *electrolyte imbalances*, particularly **hypernatremia** (high

sodium levels) and hypokalemia (low potassium levels).

2. **Alkalosis Risk:** Overuse or incorrect administration can result in *metabolic alkalosis*, where the body's pH becomes too high, leading to muscle twitching, hand tremors, and other symptoms.

3. **Gastrointestinal Side Effects:** Oral administration can cause gastrointestinal issues like bloating and gas due to the release of carbon dioxide gas when it neutralizes stomach acid.

4. **Interactions with Medications:** It can interact with various medications, altering their absorption and effectiveness, which requires careful management in patients on multiple medications.

In medical practice, the use of *sodium bicarbonate* must be carefully balanced, considering the patient's overall health, existing conditions, and potential risks associated with its use.

# Simethicone: *Simethicone* is an

over-the-counter medication widely used to relieve bloating, discomfort, and painful pressure caused by excess gas in the stomach and intestines. It is a defoaming agent that works by reducing the surface tension of gas bubbles, causing them to combine into larger bubbles that can be passed more easily from the body. This action helps to alleviate symptoms of gas such as belching, bloating, and feelings of fullness.

*Simethicone* is available in various forms, including chewable tablets, capsules, and liquid, making it accessible and easy to use for adults and children alike. It is often found in combination with other digestive aid medications to provide symptomatic relief for a range of gastrointestinal discomforts.

Importantly, simethicone does not get absorbed into the bloodstream, making it a safe option for most individuals, including pregnant and breastfeeding women, although consulting a healthcare provider is always recommended. It is generally well-tolerated, with minimal side effects, and can be taken as needed, making it a popular choice for managing gastrointestinal gas symptoms.

## Pros

1. **Effective Gas Relief:** *Simethicone* works by reducing the surface tension of gas bubbles in the stomach and intestines, making it easier for them to combine and be expelled from the body. This action can provide quick relief from bloating, discomfort, and pain associated with gas.

2. **Safe for Wide Use:** It is considered safe for most people, including pregnant women and children, when used as directed. Simethicone is not absorbed into the bloodstream, making it a low-risk option for managing gas symptoms.

3. **Compatibility with Other Medications:** Since simethicone is not absorbed by the body, it generally does not interact with other medications, making it safe to use in conjunction with other treatments.

4. **Ease of Use:** Available in various forms, such as tablets, liquid, and chewable tablets, simethicone is easy to administer and can be taken as needed, which is convenient for users.

# Cons

**Limited Scope of Effectiveness:** While effective for relieving symptoms associated with gas, *simethicone* does not treat the underlying cause of gas production. It may require concurrent treatment for conditions like *Irritable Bowel Syndrome (IBS)* or *Lactose Intolerance*.

**Possible Allergic Reactions:** Although rare, some individuals may experience allergic reactions to simethicone, including itching, swelling, or difficulty breathing.

**Not a Cure-All for Digestive Issues:** It may not be effective for all types of abdominal discomfort or bloating not caused by gas, such as those resulting from constipation or certain gastrointestinal diseases.

**Overuse Concerns:** While overuse is not typically associated with serious side effects, relying heavily on simethicone without addressing dietary or lifestyle factors that contribute to gas may not be advisable.

In summary, *simethicone* is a widely used, safe, and effective treatment for managing gastrointestinal gas, though it is important to consider its limitations and the potential need for addressing underlying causes of gas production.

# H2 Blockers

## Zantac 360°, Pepcid AC, Tagamet HB, Axid AR

*H2 blockers* (or *histamine–2 receptor antagonists*) are a class of medications used to decrease the production of stomach acid. They work by blocking the action of **histamine** on the *histamine H2 receptors* of the stomach's **parietal cells,** which are responsible for acid secretion. By inhibiting this action, *H2 blockers* effectively reduce the volume and concentration of stomach acid, providing relief from conditions like *peptic ulcers, gastroesophageal reflux disease (GERD)*, and *Zollinger–Ellison Syndrome*.

These medications are beneficial for managing symptoms of heartburn and indigestion because they can decrease the acidity of the stomach, which in turn reduces the irritation and damage that can occur when acid refluxes into the *esophagus*. They are generally considered to be faster acting than antacids but slower in onset than **Proton Pump Inhibitors (PPIs)**, with effects lasting up to 12 hours.

H2 blockers are available in both over-the-counter and prescription forms, depending on the dosage and specific needs of the patient. They are generally well-tolerated, but as with any medication, they may have side effects and interactions with other medications, so consultation with a healthcare provider is recommended before starting treatment.

Please note that availability, brand names, and regulatory status of these medications can vary by country. Additionally, some of these medications may be available under generic names or different brand names in various regions.

# H2 Blocker Medicines

Some very well known brand names that are considered H2 Blockers available for purchase. Availability may depend on your location.

**Zantac 360°:** *Zantac 360°* contains *Famotidine* as its active ingredient. *Famotidine* is an H2 (histamine-2) blocker that works by reducing the amount of acid your stomach produces. It's used for the treatment and prevention of heartburn, acid indigestion, and sour stomach. Always check the product's packaging for the most current and specific information regarding ingredients and consult with a healthcare provider if you have questions about its use.

# Pepcid AC: Almost identical to *Zantac 360°*,

Pepcid AC also is an over-the-counter medication that contains **Famotidine**. Pepcid AC is designed for short-term use and is effective in managing the symptoms of *(GERD)* and other conditions characterized by excessive stomach acid.

The medication is well-tolerated, with side effects being rare and generally mild. However, as with any medication, it's important for users to follow the recommended dosages and consult with a healthcare provider if they have any concerns about its use, especially if they are pregnant, nursing, have existing medical conditions, or are taking other medications that could potentially interact with famotidine.

# Tagamet HB: *Tagamet HB* is also an *H2*

*blocker (histamine–2 receptor antagonist)* medication but contains **Cimetidine.** A different type used to reduce the production of stomach acid. It is primarily used for the treatment and prevention of heartburn, acid indigestion, and sour stomach. Additionally, Tagamet HB can be used to treat conditions such as *gastroesophageal reflux disease (GERD)* and certain types of ulcers by decreasing the amount of acid produced in the stomach, thereby relieving symptoms associated with excessive stomach acid.

*Cimetidine*, the active ingredient in Tagamet HB, works

by blocking *histamine H2 receptors* on the cells in the stomach lining that are responsible for acid secretion.

Tagamet HB is designed for short-term use and is available without a prescription, making it a convenient option for those seeking relief from acid-related discomfort.

# Axid AR: *Axid AR* (Acid Reducer) is an additional *H2 Blocker* medication, but contains **Nizatidine**. It also is designed to prevent and relieve heartburn symptoms associated with acid indigestion and sour stomach.

*Nizatidine* works by reducing the amount of acid produced in the stomach.
Axid AR is used for the short-term treatment of heartburn and acid reflux symptoms, allowing individuals to manage these conditions with an effective, non-prescription option.

It is intended for those seeking quick relief from occasional heartburn, providing a convenient way to control stomach acid production and alleviate the burning sensation commonly experienced with acid-related digestive issues.

# H2 Blockers Medicines
## Compounds Used – Pros & Cons

Famotidine, Cimetidine, Nizatidine

**Famotidine:** *Famotidine* is a medication belonging to the class of drugs known as *H2 receptor antagonists* or *H2 blockers*. It works by reducing the amount of acid produced by the stomach, making it highly effective in treating and preventing various conditions related to excessive stomach acid. These conditions include *peptic ulcers* (both gastric and **duodenal ulcers**), *gastroesophageal reflux disease (GERD)*, and *Zollinger–Ellison syndrome*, a disorder that leads to tumors that increase acid production.

*Famotidine* is available both over-the-counter (OTC) and by prescription, depending on the dosage required. It can relieve symptoms such as heartburn, acid indigestion, and sour stomach. When used in a hospital setting, famotidine may also be administered intravenously for those who cannot take oral medications.

This medication is favored for its long action duration and fewer side effects compared to other antacids and acid reducers, like *proton pump inhibitors*. Common side effects are minimal but can include headache, dizziness, and constipation or diarrhea. Famotidine's ability to effectively manage acid production with a lower incidence of side effects makes it a popular choice for both doctors and patients in the management of acid-related gastrointestinal disorders.

## **Pros**

1. **Efficacy:** *Famotidine* is effective in reducing the production of stomach acid, providing relief from heartburn, healing ulcers, and managing *GERD* symptoms.

2. **Fast-acting:** It starts working within an hour of ingestion, offering quick relief from acid reflux and heartburn.

3. **Long Duration:** It has a longer duration of action compared to antacids, providing sustained relief.

4. **Less Frequent Dosing:** Due to its longer-lasting effects, famotidine typically requires less frequent dosing compared to antacids or some other H2 blockers.

5. **OTC Availability:** Available over the counter, it's convenient for patients to access without a prescription for the management of occasional heartburn and indigestion.

6. **Safety Profile:** Generally, famotidine is well-tolerated by most patients, with a relatively low risk of serious side effects when used as directed.

# Cons

1. **Drug Interactions:** *Famotidine* can interact with certain medications, potentially affecting their absorption and efficacy, such as certain *antifungals* and heart medications.

2. **Side Effects:** While usually mild, side effects can include headache, dizziness, constipation, or diarrhea. Rarely, more serious side effects like an irregular heartbeat or allergic reactions can occur.

3. **Not for Immediate Relief:** It may not provide the immediate relief of symptoms that antacids can, as it works by reducing acid production over time.

4. **Potential for Overuse:** Easy accessibility might lead to overuse or misuse, potentially masking symptoms of more serious conditions.

5. **Tolerance Development:** Long-term use might lead to decreased effectiveness, requiring higher doses for the same relief.

In summary, *famotidine* offers a viable option for those seeking to manage conditions associated with excess stomach acid. However, like all medications, it should be used responsibly and ideally under the guidance of a healthcare provider to ensure its benefits outweigh any potential risks.

## Cimetidine: *Cimetidine* is a medication

belonging to the class of *H2 receptor antagonists*. It works by reducing the amount of acid produced in the stomach, making it effective in the treatment and prevention of various gastrointestinal conditions such as *peptic ulcers, (GERD),* and *Zollinger–Ellison syndrome.* Introduced in the 1970s, *cimetidine* represented a significant advancement in acid-related disorder treatments, offering patients relief from the discomfort and potential complications of excessive stomach acid.

While cimetidine is effective and has been widely used, it is known for its potential to interact with a broad range of medications, affecting their metabolism and increasing the risk of side effects. Common side effects of cimetidine can include headaches, dizziness, and gastrointestinal disturbances. Despite these drawbacks, its ability to significantly improve symptoms of acid reflux and ulcers has made it a valuable tool in gastrointestinal healthcare. However, newer *H2 blockers* with fewer side effects and interactions have since become more commonly prescribed.

*Cimetidine*, marketed under the brand name Tagamet among others, is a medication that belongs to the class of *H2 receptor antagonists*. It was once a frontline treatment for *peptic ulcers*, *(GERD)*, and conditions that cause excessive stomach acid like *Zollinger–Ellison syndrome*. Despite its effectiveness, the use of cimetidine comes with both advantages and disadvantages.

## **Pros**

1. **Broad Effectiveness:** *Cimetidine* effectively reduces the production of stomach acid, providing relief from the symptoms of ulcers, *GERD*, and other acid-related disorders.

2. **Prevention of Ulcers:** It can prevent the formation of ulcers in the stomach and duodenum, especially in patients at risk due to continuous use of *NSAIDs*.

3. **Longer Duration of Action:** Compared to antacids, cimetidine offers a longer duration of acid suppression, providing prolonged relief from symptoms.

4. **Cost-Effective:** Being one of the first *H2 blockers* on the market, it is generally less

expensive than newer medications, making it a cost-effective option for many patients.

## <u>Cons</u>

1. **Drug Interactions:** *Cimetidine* can interact with a wide range of medications, potentially increasing their levels in the blood and leading to adverse effects. This is due to its ability to inhibit certain enzymes in the liver responsible for drug metabolism.

2. **Side Effects:** Possible side effects include headache, dizziness, diarrhea, and tiredness. Less commonly, it can cause more severe reactions like confusion (especially in the elderly), impotence, and **gynecomastia** (breast enlargement in men) with long-term use.

3. **Superseded by Newer Medications:** Newer $H2$ *blockers* and *proton pump inhibitors (PPIs)* with fewer side effects and interactions have largely superseded cimetidine in clinical use.

4. **Requires Multiple Daily Doses:** For effective management of symptoms, cimetidine often needs to be taken multiple times a day, which can be less convenient compared to once-daily medications like *PPIs*.

While *cimetidine* has been a pivotal medication in the treatment of acid-related disorders, its use has declined in favor of drugs with better safety profiles, fewer drug interactions, and more convenient dosing schedules.

# Nizatidine: *Nizatidine* is a medication that falls under the category of *H2 receptor antagonists*, similar to *famotidine* and *cimetidine*. It functions by inhibiting the action of *histamine* on the stomach's parietal cells, thereby decreasing the production of stomach acid. This reduction in acid can effectively treat and prevent ulcers in the stomach and intestines, as well as manage conditions such as *(GERD)*, where acid from the stomach flows back into the *esophagus*, causing heartburn and potential injury to the esophageal lining.

Introduced for medical use in the 1980s, *nizatidine* has been appreciated for its efficacy and relatively favorable safety profile, with common side effects being mild and including headache, dizziness, and gastrointestinal disturbances. Its once-daily dosing convenience made it a preferred choice for patients seeking relief from acid-related discomfort. However, like other *H2 blockers*, it's essential to use nizatidine judiciously and under medical guidance to avoid potential drug interactions and ensure its benefits are maximized.

# **<u>Pros</u>**

1. **Efficacy:** *Nizatidine* effectively reduces stomach acid production, which can alleviate symptoms of heartburn, acid reflux, and promote the healing of ulcers.

2. **Rapid Action:** It begins to reduce acid production within an hour of ingestion, providing relatively quick relief from symptoms.

3. **Fewer Central Nervous System Side Effects:** Compared to other *H2 blockers* like *cimetidine*, *nizatidine* has a lower risk of crossing the blood-brain barrier, which means it is less likely to cause central nervous system side effects such as confusion, especially in elderly patients.

4. **Minimal Drug Interactions:** Nizatidine has fewer drug interactions than cimetidine, making it a safer option for patients taking multiple medications.

5. **Once-Daily Dosing:** It can often be taken once daily, which improves convenience and adherence to treatment.

# <u>Cons</u>

1. **Side Effects:** While generally well-tolerated, *nizatidine* can cause side effects such as headache, dizziness, diarrhea, or constipation in some patients.

2. **Limited Effectiveness for Severe Cases:** For severe cases of *GERD* or ulcers, nizatidine may not be as effective as *proton pump inhibitors (PPIs)*, which more profoundly suppress stomach acid production.

3. **Potential for Drug Interactions:** Despite having fewer interactions than some other *H2 blockers*, nizatidine can still interact with certain drugs, affecting their absorption and efficacy.

4. **Kidney Function Monitoring:** In patients with renal impairment, dose adjustments may be necessary, requiring monitoring of kidney function.

5. **Withdrawal from Market:** As of my last update, nizatidine had been withdrawn from the market in some countries due to contamination concerns, which may limit its availability.

In summary, *nizatidine* offers a beneficial option for treating conditions associated with excessive stomach acid, with a relatively favorable side effect and interaction profile. However, considerations regarding its effectiveness, side effects, and current availability are essential when choosing it as a treatment option.

# Proton Pump Inhibitors (PPI)

## Prilosec, Nexium, Prevacid, Protonix, Aciphex, Dexilant

*Proton Pump Inhibitors (PPIs)* are a class of medications widely used to treat conditions associated with excessive stomach acid production, such as *gastroesophageal reflux disease (GERD), peptic ulcers, and Zollinger–Ellison syndrome. PPIs* are among the most potent inhibitors of acid secretion available. They work by irreversibly blocking the **hydrogen–potassium ATPase enzyme system** (the proton pump) on the surface of the gastric parietal cells. This action effectively stops the final step in the production of *gastric acid*, significantly reducing the amount of acid in the stomach.

The reduction in stomach acid provides relief from the symptoms of acid reflux, such as heartburn and indigestion, and allows for the healing of ulcers and inflammation in the *esophagus* or stomach. *PPIs* are more effective and have a longer duration of action than other acid-reducing medications, such as *H2 blockers*, making them a preferred choice for long-term management of acid-related disorders.

These medications are available in both over-the-counter and prescription forms. While *PPIs* are generally well-tolerated, long-term use has been associated with several potential risks, including **nutrient malabsorption** and increased susceptibility to infections. Therefore, their use should be carefully considered and monitored by healthcare professionals.

# Proton Pump Inhibitor Medicines

A few very popular brand names identified as Proton Pump Inhibitors (PPIs) medications available in most drug stores. Their availability may differ depending on your regional area.

## Prilosec: *Prilosec's* active ingredient is

*Omeprazole*. It works by blocking the *enzyme* in the stomach lining responsible for acid secretion, providing relief from symptoms like heartburn, regurgitation, and difficulty swallowing.
Available over-the-counter and by prescription, it's recommended for short-term treatment of ulcers and *GERD*, and in combination with antibiotics for certain gastric infections.

*Omeprazole* is used to treat various conditions related to excess stomach acid, including *(GERD)*, *peptic ulcers*, and *Zollinger–Ellison syndrome*. By decreasing stomach acid production, it helps alleviate symptoms such as heartburn, acid reflux, and promotes healing of the esophagus and stomach.

Prilosec is available in different formulations, including delayed-release capsules and over-the-counter tablets, which are designed to ensure that the medication is released into the body at the right time to maximize its effectiveness while minimizing potential side effects. Always consult a healthcare professional for appropriate diagnosis and treatment options tailored to individual health needs.

While Prilosec is widely regarded for its effectiveness in managing acid-related disorders, patients should consult healthcare professionals before starting the medication to discuss potential side effects and long-term use implications.

## Nexium: *Nexium*, scientifically known as *esomeprazole*, is also a *proton pump inhibitor (PPI)* widely used in the treatment of *(GERD)*. *Esomeprazole* works by blocking the *enzyme* in the wall of the stomach that produces acid, thereby reducing the amount of acid in the stomach. This mechanism helps in the healing of acid-related damage to the lining of the *esophagus* and prevents ulcers in the stomach and intestines.

Nexium is also prescribed for treating *Zollinger–Ellison syndrome*, a disorder marked by the excessive production of stomach acid, and for the prevention of **gastric ulcers** caused by the prolonged use of nonsteroidal anti-inflammatory drugs *(NSAIDs)* or infection with *Helicobacter pylori*. Additionally, it may be used in combination with antibiotics to treat certain types of *gastric ulcers*.

Available in both over-the-counter and prescription strengths, Nexium is taken orally, typically once a day, about one hour before meals. While it is effective in reducing acid and alleviating symptoms associated with acid reflux, long-term use of Nexium and other *PPIs* has been associated with various potential side effects, including vitamin B12 deficiency, kidney issues, and increased risk of bone fractures. Patients are advised to use the lowest effective dose for the shortest duration necessary to manage their symptoms.

## Prevacid: *Prevacid*, known generically as *Lansoprazole*, is a *proton pump inhibitor (PPI)* medication designed to reduce the amount of acid produced in the stomach. It is primarily used to treat and prevent stomach and intestinal ulcers, erosive *esophagitis* (damage to the esophagus from stomach acid), and other conditions involving excessive stomach acid such as *Zollinger–Ellison syndrome*. Prevacid is

also commonly prescribed for the management of (GERD), a condition causing heartburn and potential injury to the esophageal lining.

By inhibiting the action of the proton pumps in the stomach lining, Prevacid effectively decreases the level of acid in the stomach, which helps in healing acid-damaged tissues and prevents ulcers and inflammation. This makes it a valuable treatment option for those suffering from acid-related gastrointestinal conditions.

Prevacid is available over the counter and by prescription, and it comes in various forms, including capsules, orally disintegrating tablets, and as a liquid suspension. While Prevacid is effective in relieving symptoms associated with excessive stomach acid, long-term use has been linked to potential side effects, such as vitamin B12 deficiency, magnesium deficiency, and an increased risk of bone fractures. Patients are advised to discuss the benefits and risks of long-term Prevacid use with their healthcare provider.

**Protonix:** *Protonix*, with the generic name *Pantoprazole*, is another  medication classified as a *proton pump inhibitor (PPI)* used to treat certain stomach and *esophagus* problems, such as acid reflux and ***erosive esophagitis***. It works by reducing the amount of acid produced in the stomach, providing relief from symptoms like heartburn, difficulty swallowing, and persistent cough. This action not only helps heal acid damage to the stomach and *esophagus* but also prevents ulcers and may prevent cancer of the esophagus. Protonix is commonly prescribed for the treatment of *gastroesophageal reflux disease (GERD)* and conditions involving excessive stomach acid production, such as *Zollinger–Ellison syndrome.*

Pantoprazole is typically taken by mouth, in either tablet or liquid form, and is available both over the counter and by prescription. Patients are advised to follow their healthcare provider's instructions closely when taking Protonix, as the dosage and duration of treatment can vary based on the condition being treated.

While Protonix is effective in managing symptoms associated with acid-related disorders, long-term use has been associated with potential risks, including vitamin B12 deficiency, magnesium deficiency, and an increased risk of bone fractures, especially with high doses or prolonged use. As with any medication, it's important for patients to discuss the potential benefits and risks of using Protonix with their healthcare provider, ensuring it aligns with their overall treatment plan.

**Aciphex:** *Aciphex*, whose generic name is *Rabeprazole*, is an additional *proton pump inhibitor (PPIs)*. It is prescribed for the treatment of several gastrointestinal conditions including heartburn, *(GERD)*, and injury to the esophageal lining. Aciphex is also effective in healing *erosive esophagitis* (damage to the esophagus from stomach acid) and in treating conditions that lead to excessive stomach acid, such as *Zollinger–Ellison syndrome*.

*Rabeprazole* works by blocking the enzyme in the stomach wall that produces acid, thereby reducing the amount of acid in the stomach. This decrease in stomach acid allows the *esophagus* and stomach to heal from acid-related damage and prevents the formation of ulcers.

Available by prescription, Aciphex is usually taken once daily, with or without food. While it is effective in managing symptoms and promoting healing, long-term use of Aciphex, as with other *PPIs*, may be associated with certain risks, including vitamin B12 deficiency, magnesium deficiency, and an increased risk of fractures. Therefore, it is important for patients to discuss the potential benefits and risks of using Aciphex with their healthcare provider.

**Dexilant:** *Dexilant*, known generically as *Dexlansoprazole*, is a *proton pump inhibitor (PPI)* medication designed to treat *gastroesophageal reflux disease (GERD)* and related conditions. It is specifically aimed at relieving symptoms such as heartburn, difficulty swallowing, and persistent cough that result from stomach acid flowing back into the esophagus. Dexilant works by reducing the amount of acid produced in the stomach, offering relief from the discomfort associated with acid reflux and aiding in the healing of acid-related damage to the throat and *esophagus*.

One of the unique features of Dexilant is its dual delayed-release formulation, which allows it to provide two separate releases of medication. This results in an extended period of acid suppression, offering improved symptom management over a longer duration compared to some other *PPIs*. Dexilant is typically prescribed for once-daily use, and it can be taken with or without food.

While Dexilant is effective in managing *GERD* symptoms and promoting healing in the *esophagus*, long-term use of this and other *PPIs* has been linked to potential side effects, including risks of vitamin B12 deficiency, magnesium deficiency, and increased risk of bone fractures. Patients considering Dexilant should consult with their healthcare provider to weigh the benefits and risks, ensuring it aligns with their overall health management plan.

These brand names represent the most commonly used *PPIs*. The specific brand available and whether it requires a prescription can depend on the regulatory environment of the country in which you are located.

*PPIs* are highly effective in reducing stomach acid secretion by directly inhibiting the enzyme system responsible for acid production in the stomach, offering relief from acid-related symptoms and promoting healing of the esophagus and stomach in conditions like *GERD* and ulcers.

Always consult a healthcare provider for the appropriate selection and use of PPIs, as they can advise on the best treatment plan based on individual health needs.

# Proton Pump Inhibitors (PPI)
## Compounds Used – Pros & Cons

Omeprazole, Esomeprazole, Lansoprazole, Pantoprazole, Rabeprazole, Dexlansoprazole

**Omeprazole:** *Omeprazole* is a widely used medication belonging to the class of drugs known as *proton pump inhibitors (PPIs)*. Its primary function is to reduce the production of stomach acid, making it an effective treatment for conditions related to excess acid such as *(GERD)*, ulcers, and *Zollinger–Ellison syndrome*. By inhibiting the enzyme in the wall of the stomach that produces acid, omeprazole allows for the healing of damaged esophageal tissue, relieves symptoms of heartburn, and prevents ulcers.

It's also used in combination with antibiotics to treat certain types of stomach ulcers caused by *Helicobacter pylori bacteria*. Omeprazole is available in both over-the-counter and prescription strengths, and it is taken orally in the form of capsules or tablets.

While omeprazole is generally well-tolerated, long-term use may lead to side effects such as vitamin B12 deficiency, kidney problems, and an increased risk of bone fractures. It's important for patients to use this medication under the guidance of a healthcare provider to manage conditions effectively while minimizing potential risks.

## Pros

1. **Effective Acid Suppression:** *Omeprazole* effectively reduces stomach acid production, which is beneficial for treating acid-related conditions such as *GERD, peptic ulcers, and Zollinger–Ellison syndrome.*

2. **Symptom Relief:** It provides relief from symptoms associated with excess stomach acid, such as heartburn, acid reflux, and indigestion.

3. **Healing of Esophageal Damage:** By reducing acid production, omeprazole can help heal damage to the *esophagus* caused by acid reflux.

4. **Prevention of Ulcers:** It is used to prevent the formation of ulcers, especially in individuals taking *NSAIDs* for long periods.

5. **Treatment of H. pylori Infections:** In combination with antibiotics, omeprazole is effective in treating stomach ulcers caused by **H. pylori infections.**

# <u>Cons</u>

1. **Risk of Chronic Kidney Disease:** Long-term use of *omeprazole* has been associated with an increased risk of chronic kidney disease.

2. **Bone Fracture Risk:** Extended use may lead to decreased calcium absorption, potentially increasing the risk of bone fractures, especially in the elderly or those with osteoporosis.

3. **Vitamin B12 Deficiency:** Prolonged use can reduce the absorption of vitamin B12, leading to deficiency, particularly in the elderly or those with existing nutritional deficiencies.

4. **Clostridium difficile Infection:** There is an increased risk of *Clostridium difficile infection* in the gut, which can lead to severe diarrhea and *Colitis*, associated with long-term *PPI* use.

5. **Drug Interactions:** Omeprazole can interact with other medications, affecting their absorption and efficacy, such as certain antifungals, antiplatelets, and HIV medications.

It's essential for individuals considering omeprazole for treatment to consult with healthcare providers. This ensures that the benefits outweigh the risks, especially for long-term use. Adjustments in dosage and monitoring for potential side effects are crucial aspects of managing treatment with omeprazole effectively.

**Esomeprazole:** *Esomeprazole,* is an additional *proton pump inhibitor (PPI)* used to reduce stomach acid production. It is the *S-isomer* **of** *omeprazole* (see Glossary for more info), offering a more targeted form for treating acid-related gastrointestinal conditions. *Esomeprazole* is primarily prescribed for the management of *(GERD)*, where it alleviates symptoms such as heartburn and prevents the damage to the *esophagus* caused by stomach acid. It is also effective in healing erosive *esophagitis* and in the treatment of conditions like *Zollinger-Ellison syndrome,* which involve excessive acid production in the stomach.

*Esomeprazole* is beneficial in preventing ulcers caused by *non-steroidal anti-inflammatory drugs (NSAIDs)* and in the eradication of *Helicobacter Pylori Bacteria* when used in combination with antibiotics. Available in oral and intravenous forms, it is often chosen for its efficacy in acid suppression and symptom relief. However, similar to other *PPIs,* long-term use of esomeprazole can lead to potential side effects, including risks of vitamin B12 deficiency, bone fractures, kidney issues, and increased susceptibility to infections like *Clostridium difficile.*

Despite these concerns, *esomeprazole* remains a valuable tool in managing acid-related disorders, with its use tailored to individual needs under medical guidance.

## Pros

1. **Effective Acid Suppression:** *Esomeprazole* is highly effective in reducing stomach acid, making it beneficial for treating conditions like *GERD, peptic ulcers, and Zollinger–Ellison syndrome.*

2. **Symptom Relief:** It provides significant relief from symptoms such as heartburn, acid reflux, and indigestion, improving quality of life for patients with acid-related disorders.

3. **Healing of Esophageal Damage:** Esomeprazole helps in healing *erosive esophagitis* and other damage to the esophagus caused by acid reflux, preventing complications.

4. **Ulcer Prevention:** It is used to prevent *gastric ulcers* associated with the use of *NSAIDs* and to treat ulcers caused by *H. pylori infection* when combined with antibiotics.

5. **Once-Daily Dosing:** Its formulation allows for once-daily dosing, which can improve patient compliance compared to medications requiring multiple doses per day.

# <u>Cons</u>

1. **Risk of Kidney Issues:** Long-term use has been associated with an increased risk of chronic kidney disease and acute kidney injury.

2. **Bone Fracture Risk:** Prolonged use can lead to a higher risk of bone fractures, particularly in the hip, wrist, and spine, due to potential calcium absorption impairment.

3. **Nutritional Deficiencies:** There's a risk of vitamin B12, magnesium, and possibly iron deficiency with long-term use, as stomach acid is necessary for the absorption of these nutrients.

4. **Infection Risk:** Increased risk of gastrointestinal infections, including *Clostridium difficile*, and possibly other respiratory infections due to altered stomach pH affecting the gut microbiome.

5. **Drug Interactions:** Esomeprazole can interact with other drugs, affecting how they work or how well esomeprazole works, which requires careful management of medication regimens.

While *esomeprazole* is an effective treatment for managing acid-related gastrointestinal conditions, its long-term use necessitates careful consideration of the potential risks and side effects. Patients should be closely monitored by healthcare providers to ensure the benefits outweigh the risks, especially with prolonged therapy.

**Lansoprazole:** *Lansoprazole* is another *proton pump inhibitor (PPI)* medication used to decrease the amount of acid produced in the stomach. Commonly prescribed for the treatment of *(GERD)*, *peptic ulcers,* and *Zollinger–Ellison syndrome. Lansoprazole* works by inhibiting the proton pump in the stomach lining, a mechanism crucial for acid secretion. This action provides relief from symptoms like heartburn, difficulty swallowing, and persistent cough.

Additionally, it aids in healing acid-related damage to the digestive system and prevents the formation of ulcers, especially in patients taking *NSAIDs* that can harm the stomach lining. *Lansoprazole* is also utilized in combination with antibiotics to eradicate *Helicobacter pylori bacteria*, a common cause of ulcer disease. Available in capsule form or as a disintegrating tablet, *lansoprazole* offers flexibility in administration. Despite its effectiveness, long-term use may lead to potential side effects, including vitamin B12 deficiency, bone fractures, and an increased risk of infections.

# Pros

1. **Effective Acid Control:** *Lansoprazole* efficiently reduces stomach acid, providing relief from symptoms of acid reflux, *GERD*, and conditions like *peptic ulcers* and *Zollinger–Ellison syndrome.*

2. **Symptom Relief and Healing:** It aids in the relief of symptoms such as heartburn and indigestion, and promotes the healing of the *esophagus* and stomach lining damaged by excess acid.

3. **Ulcer Prevention:** It is effective in preventing ulcers, especially in individuals who are at risk due to the long-term use of *NSAIDs.*

4. **Treatment of H. pylori:** When used in combination with antibiotics, lansoprazole helps in eradicating *H. pylori bacteria,* a common cause of ulcers.

5. **Flexible Dosage Forms:** Available in capsule and orally disintegrating tablet forms, it offers options for patients who have difficulty swallowing pills.

# <u>Cons</u>

1. **Kidney Issues:** Long-term use has been linked with an increased risk of chronic kidney disease and acute kidney injury.

2. **Bone Fracture Risk:** Extended use may lead to a higher risk of bone fractures, possibly due to impaired calcium absorption.

3. **Nutritional Deficiencies:** There is a potential for deficiencies in vitamin B12, magnesium, and iron with prolonged use, as stomach acid is necessary for the absorption of these nutrients.

4. **Infection Risk:** Increased susceptibility to gastrointestinal infections, such as *Clostridium difficile*, and possibly respiratory infections, due to changes in stomach pH and *microbiome*.

5. **Drug Interactions:** Lansoprazole can interact with other medications, affecting how they are absorbed and metabolized, which could diminish their efficacy or increase side effects.

The use of *lansoprazole*, like other *PPIs*, should be carefully considered, balancing its benefits in managing acid-related conditions against the potential risks, especially with long-term therapy. Monitoring and consultation with a healthcare provider are essential to optimize treatment outcomes and minimize adverse effects.

# **Pantoprazole:** *Pantoprazole,* a *proton pump inhibitor (PPI)* that significantly reduces stomach acid production, making it an effective treatment for various acid-related gastrointestinal disorders. It is commonly prescribed for conditions like *gastroesophageal reflux disease (GERD),* where it helps manage symptoms such as heartburn and acid reflux, and for the healing of *erosive esophagitis. Pantoprazole* is also used in the treatment and prevention of stomach and *duodenal ulcers,* including those induced by the use of *non-steroidal anti-inflammatory drugs (NSAIDs).* Furthermore, it can be part of the therapy for *Zollinger-Ellison syndrome,* a condition characterized by excessive acid production.

Administered orally or intravenously, *pantoprazole* offers flexibility in treatment, particularly for patients unable to take oral medication. Despite its effectiveness in managing acid-related conditions, long-term use of pantoprazole may be associated with potential risks such as vitamin B12 deficiency, bone fractures, kidney issues, and an increased risk of certain infections. Therefore, its use should be carefully monitored by healthcare professionals to balance the benefits against potential side effects.

# Pros

1. **Effective Acid Suppression:** *Pantoprazole* is highly effective at reducing stomach acid, aiding in the treatment of *GERD, peptic ulcers, and Zollinger–Ellison syndrome.*

2. **Symptom Relief:** It offers relief from symptoms such as heartburn, acid reflux, and indigestion, improving patients' quality of life.

3. **Healing Esophageal Damage:** By reducing acid production, pantoprazole promotes healing of damage to the *esophagus* caused by acid reflux, preventing further complications.

4. **Prevention of Ulcers:** It is effective in preventing ulcers, especially in patients at risk due to the long-term use of *NSAIDs*.

5. **Flexibility in Administration:** Available in oral and intravenous forms, pantoprazole provides treatment options for patients unable to take pills.

# Cons

1. **Kidney Issues:** Long-term use has been linked to an increased risk of ***chronic kidney disease*** and acute kidney injury.

2. **Bone Fracture Risk:** Prolonged use may increase the risk of bone fractures, potentially due to decreased calcium absorption.

3. **Nutritional Deficiencies:** Extended use can lead to deficiencies in vitamin B12, magnesium, and possibly iron, as stomach acid is crucial for their absorption.

4. **Risk of Infections:** There is an increased risk of *Clostridium difficile infection* in the gut and possibly other respiratory infections due to alterations in stomach pH and *flora*.

5. **Drug Interactions:** Pantoprazole can interact with other medications, potentially affecting their effectiveness or how well pantoprazole works.

The use of pantoprazole necessitates a careful balance between its benefits in controlling acid-related symptoms and the potential risks associated with long-term therapy.

Regular monitoring and consultation with a healthcare provider are essential to ensure that the medication's use is optimized for the individual's health needs.

# **Rabeprazole:** *Rabeprazole* is a *proton pump inhibitor (PPI)* that decreases the amount of acid produced in the stomach, used extensively in the treatment of gastrointestinal conditions related to excessive acid production. It is effective in managing symptoms and promoting healing in disorders such as (GERD), *peptic ulcers*, and conditions like *Zollinger–Ellison syndrome*. *Rabeprazole* works by blocking the enzyme in the stomach wall responsible for acid secretion, thus providing relief from discomfort such as heartburn and aiding in the healing of acid-related damage to the digestive tract.

Additionally, rabeprazole is used in combination with antibiotics in the treatment of *Helicobacter pylori infection*, a common cause of ulcers. Available in oral form, it is appreciated for its once-daily dosing convenience. While generally well-tolerated, long-term use of rabeprazole, as with other *PPIs*, may lead to potential side effects including nutrient deficiencies, increased risk of bone fractures, and susceptibility to infections. It's crucial for its use to be carefully monitored by healthcare professionals to mitigate these risks effectively.

## Pros

1. **Effective Acid Reduction:** Rabeprazole effectively decreases stomach acid production,

providing relief from conditions like *GERD, peptic ulcers, and Zollinger–Ellison syndrome.*

2. **Symptom Management:** It helps manage and alleviate symptoms such as heartburn, acid reflux, and discomfort associated with excess stomach acid.

3. **Healing of Damage:** By reducing acid levels, rabeprazole aids in the healing of the *esophagus* and stomach lining damaged by acid erosion, preventing further complications.

4. **Prevention of Ulcers:** It is effective in preventing ulcers, particularly in patients who are at risk from the long-term use of *NSAIDs.*

5. **H. pylori Eradication:** When used in combination with antibiotics, rabeprazole helps eradicate *H. pylori bacteria,* addressing one of the primary causes of ulcers.

## Cons

1. **Kidney Issues:** Long-term use has been associated with an increased risk of kidney issues, including chronic kidney disease and *acute interstitial nephritis.*

2. **Bone Fracture Risk:** Prolonged use may lead to a higher risk of bone fractures, as acid suppression can affect calcium absorption and bone health.

3. **Nutritional Deficiencies:** There's a risk of deficiencies in vitamin B12, magnesium, and iron due to reduced stomach acid, which is necessary for the absorption of these nutrients.

4. **Infection Risk:** Increased susceptibility to gastrointestinal infections, such as *Clostridium difficile*, and possibly respiratory infections, due to alterations in the stomach's acidic environment.

5. **Drug Interactions:** Rabeprazole can interact with other medications, affecting their absorption and metabolism, which could potentially reduce their efficacy or increase side effects.

While *rabeprazole* is an effective medication for managing acid-related conditions, its long-term use requires careful consideration and monitoring to balance the therapeutic benefits against potential risks. It's important for individuals to work closely with their healthcare provider to ensure the optimal use of rabeprazole in their treatment regimen.

**Dexlansoprazole:** *Dexlansoprazole* is a *proton pump inhibitor (PPI)* designed to reduce stomach acid production through a unique dual-release mechanism, offering extended and more consistent acid control compared to traditional *PPIs*. It is primarily used to treat *gastroesophageal reflux disease (GERD)*, including the healing of *erosive esophagitis* and maintenance of healed *esophagitis*, as well as to manage symptoms of heartburn. *Dexlansoprazole* works by inhibiting the proton pumps in the stomach lining responsible for acid secretion.

This dual-release formulation allows for a portion of the medication to be released immediately and another portion to be released later, providing a longer duration of acid suppression over 24 hours with a single dose. While dexlansoprazole is effective in managing acid-related disorders and is generally well-tolerated, long-term use may carry risks similar to other *PPIs*, such as vitamin B12 deficiency, bone fractures, and an increased risk of infections. It's important for patients to use dexlansoprazole under the guidance of a healthcare provider to ensure its benefits outweigh any potential risks.

## Pros

1. **Extended Acid Suppression:** The dual-release mechanism provides two phases of medication

release, offering longer and more consistent acid suppression over 24 hours, which is particularly beneficial for managing *GERD* symptoms and healing *erosive esophagitis*.

2. **Symptom Relief:** It effectively relieves symptoms associated with acid reflux, such as heartburn, providing significant improvement in quality of life for patients.

3. **Healing of Erosive Esophagitis:** *Dexlansoprazole* is highly effective in the healing and maintenance of healed *erosive esophagitis*, reducing the risk of recurrence.

4. **Convenient Dosing:** The extended release allows for once-daily dosing, which can improve patient compliance and ease of use compared to medications requiring multiple doses per day.

5. **Safety Profile:** It is generally well-tolerated by patients, with a side effect profile similar to other *PPIs*.

## <u>Cons</u>

1. **Potential for Side Effects:** Like other *PPIs*, long-term use of *dexlansoprazole* may be associated with side effects such as vitamin B12 deficiency, magnesium deficiency, and an

increased risk of bone fractures due to decreased calcium absorption.

2. **Kidney Issues:** There is a potential increased risk of chronic kidney disease and *acute interstitial nephritis* with long-term use.

3. **Infection Risks:** Increased risk of *Clostridium difficile* infection and possibly other gastrointestinal and respiratory infections due to alterations in stomach acid levels, affecting the gut microbiome.

4. **Cost:** Being a newer medication, dexlansoprazole may be more expensive than older *PPIs*, which could affect accessibility for some patients.

5. **Drug Interactions:** As with other *PPIs*, dexlansoprazole can interact with other medications, potentially affecting their efficacy or increasing the risk of adverse effects.

The decision to use *dexlansoprazole* should consider these pros and cons, balancing its benefits in managing acid-related conditions against the potential risks, especially with prolonged therapy.

# Prokinetics
## Reglan, Motilium, Zelnorm, Motegrity, Gasmotin

*Prokinetics* are a class of medication that enhances *gastrointestinal motility*, meaning they help move food and waste through the digestive system more effectively. These drugs are commonly used to treat conditions such as *gastroesophageal reflux disease (GERD)*, *gastroparesis* (delayed gastric emptying), and **chronic constipation**. By stimulating the muscles of the *gastrointestinal tract*, prokinetics can increase the rate at which the stomach empties into the intestines and speed up the movement of food through the gut.

The mechanism of action of *prokinetics* involves the stimulation of various receptors in the digestive tract, leading to increased muscle contractions. For example, some prokinetics activate **serotonin receptors**, which can enhance **motility** and the release of **acetylcholine**, a neurotransmitter that stimulates muscle contractions. Others may work by blocking dopamine receptors, which can also increase *gastrointestinal motility* since dopamine typically has an inhibitory effect on gastrointestinal movement.

In addition to their effects on motility, some prokinetics have *antiemetic* properties, meaning they can help reduce nausea and vomiting. This makes them particularly useful for conditions like *gastroparesis*, where delayed gastric emptying can lead to significant nausea and vomiting. However, prokinetics must be used carefully, as they can have side effects and are not suitable for all patients, particularly those with certain types of heart conditions or other specific health issues.

# Prokinetic Medicines

Several brand names recognized as prokinetic medications are available for purchase, although their availability might vary based on your geographical location.

**Reglan:** *Reglan* known generically as *metoclopramide*, primarily contains *metoclopramide hydrochloride* as its active ingredient. *Metoclopramide* is a *dopamine receptor antagonist* that is used to treat certain conditions of the stomach and intestines. It is effective in stimulating stomach muscle contractions to help with the movement of food through the stomach and intestines, making it useful for treating *gastroparesis* (slow stomach emptying) and for preventing nausea and vomiting associated with chemotherapy or surgery.

In addition to *metoclopramide hydrochloride*, Reglan tablets and other formulations (such as the injectable form) may include various inactive ingredients or excipients. These can include substances like **lactose, magnesium stearate, microcrystalline cellulose, and sodium starch glycolate**, among others, which are used to enhance the medication's stability, absorption, and patient tolerability. The exact composition of these inactive ingredients may vary depending on the formulation and manufacturer of the medication. It's important to consult the product's packaging or leaflet for a detailed list of ingredients, especially for individuals with allergies or sensitivities to certain compounds.

## Motilium: *Motilium* known generically as *domperidone*, is primarily composed of domperidone as its active ingredient. Domperidone is a *dopamine antagonist* with *antiemetic* properties, used to relieve symptoms of nausea and vomiting, and to treat *gastric motility* disorders such as *gastroparesis*. It works by blocking **dopamine receptors** in the brain and gut, enhancing **gastrointestinal peristalsis** and facilitating gastric emptying, without crossing the blood-brain barrier to a significant extent, which minimizes central nervous system side effects.

In addition to the active ingredient, *domperidone*, Motilium tablets and other formulations (such as suspension) may contain various excipients or inactive ingredients. These can include lactose, maize starch, microcrystalline cellulose, povidone, magnesium stearate, and sodium lauryl sulfate, among others, which are used to improve the medication's stability, absorption, and ease of administration. The specific composition of inactive ingredients may vary between different forms of the medication and different manufacturers. Always check the product leaflet for a complete list of ingredients, especially if you have allergies or sensitivities to specific excipients.

# Motegrity: *Motegrity* known generically as prucalopride, contains **prucalopride succinate** as its active ingredient. *Prucalopride* is a selective *serotonin type 4 (5–HT4) receptor agonist* that is used to treat **chronic idiopathic constipation (CIC)** in adults. It works by stimulating the muscles of the gut, enhancing bowel movements and improving symptoms of constipation.

In addition to *prucalopride succinate*, Motegrity tablets may include various inactive ingredients or excipients to ensure the stability, absorption, and ease of administration of the medication. These inactive ingredients can include but are not limited to microcrystalline cellulose, lactose monohydrate, colloidal silicon dioxide, magnesium stearate, and hypromellose. The specific composition of these excipients might vary depending on the formulation and the manufacturer.

For individuals with allergies or sensitivities, it's important to consult the product's packaging or accompanying leaflet for a detailed list of ingredients. This is especially crucial for those who need to avoid certain substances due to allergic reactions or other health concerns.

**Gasmotin:** *Gasmotin* is a brand name for the medication known generically as *Mosapride Citrate*. *Mosapride citrate* is the active ingredient in Gasmotin, which is a *gastroprokinetic agent*. It works by stimulating *serotonin 5-HT4 receptors*, enhancing *gastrointestinal motility*, and is primarily used to treat symptoms of functional *dyspepsia* and conditions such as *gastroesophageal reflux disease (GERD)* by facilitating the movement of food through the stomach and improving gastric emptying.

In addition to the active ingredient *mosapride citrate*, Gasmotin tablets may contain various inactive ingredients or excipients, which can include substances like lactose, magnesium stearate, microcrystalline cellulose, and others depending on the formulation. These excipients help in the manufacturing process, improve the stability of the medication, and enhance its absorption and usability.

The specific composition of these inactive ingredients might vary between different formulations and manufacturers of mosapride. For detailed information on the compounds in a specific product, it's important to consult the product's packaging or accompanying leaflet, especially for individuals with allergies or sensitivities to certain substances.

# Prokinetic Medicines
## Compounds Used – Pros & Cons

Metoclopramide, Domperidone, Prucalopride Succinate, Mosapride Citrate

**Metoclopramide:** *Metoclopramide* is a medication that serves as a *prokinetic* agent, specifically designed to improve *gastrointestinal motility*, which is the movement of food through the stomach and intestines. It is primarily used to treat *(GERD)*, *gastroparesis* (particularly in diabetic patients), and as an *antiemetic* to prevent nausea and vomiting associated with chemotherapy, postoperative states, and other medical conditions.

*Metoclopramide* works by antagonizing *dopamine receptors* in the gastrointestinal tract and the brain's **chemoreceptor trigger zone**, leading to enhanced gastric emptying and increased lower *esophageal sphincter* tone. This action helps reduce reflux symptoms and accelerates the transit of food through the stomach.

The drug is available in various formulations, including oral (tablets and liquid) and injectable forms, allowing for versatile use in both outpatient and inpatient settings. Despite its effectiveness in improving *gastrointestinal motility* and providing *antiemetic* benefits, metoclopramide's use must be carefully monitored due to its potential side effects. Common adverse effects include fatigue, dizziness, and **somnolence**. More serious concerns involve neurological side effects, such as **Tardive Dyskinesia**—a condition characterized by irreversible, involuntary, repetitive movements of the face and body. The risk of such neurological side effects increases with long-term use and in older patients.

Given these considerations, metoclopramide is recommended for short-term use, typically not exceeding 12 weeks, to minimize the risk of severe side effects. Healthcare providers must evaluate the benefits and risks of metoclopramide therapy on an individual basis, considering the specific needs and health conditions of each patient. This careful approach ensures that the therapeutic advantages of metoclopramide in enhancing gastrointestinal motility and controlling nausea and vomiting are balanced against the potential for adverse effects.

# Pros

1. **Effective Antiemetic:** *Metoclopramide* is highly effective at preventing nausea and vomiting, including that induced by chemotherapy, radiation, and postoperative states, improving patients' comfort and quality of life.

2. **Gastrointestinal Motility Enhancement:** By stimulating gastric emptying and intestinal motility, it helps manage symptoms of *gastroparesis* and *GERD*, such as heartburn and discomfort.

3. **Versatile Administration:** Available in oral, injectable, and intravenous forms, metoclopramide offers flexibility in administration based on patient needs and clinical settings.

4. **Rapid Onset of Action:** It works relatively quickly, making it beneficial for acute management of nausea and *gastroparesis* symptoms.

# Cons

1. **Neurological Side Effects:** *Metoclopramide* can cause ***extrapyramidal symptoms***, such as ***Tardive Dyskinesia***, especially with long-term use

or high doses. These effects may be irreversible in some cases.

2. **Restrictions on Long-term Use:** Due to the risk of neurological side effects, its use is generally recommended for short-term treatment (usually up to 12 weeks).

3. **Contraindications and Cautions:** It may not be suitable for patients with certain conditions, like Parkinson's disease, due to its *dopamine antagonist* effects.

4. **Other Side Effects:** Patients may experience other adverse effects, including fatigue, drowsiness, and diarrhea, which can affect compliance and overall well-being.

The decision to use *metoclopramide* must balance its potential benefits in improving gastrointestinal function and preventing nausea against the risk of side effects, particularly neurological ones. It necessitates careful patient selection, dosing considerations, and monitoring by healthcare professionals to ensure its safe and effective use.

**Domperidone:** *Domperidone* is a medication primarily used as a *prokinetic* agent to enhance *gastrointestinal motility*, making it particularly effective in the treatment of *gastroparesis*, nausea, and vomiting. Unlike many other prokinetic drugs, domperidone works by blocking *dopamine receptors* in the gut and the *chemoreceptor trigger zone* in the brain, which are areas that, when activated, can lead to vomiting. This mechanism facilitates gastric emptying and reduces the risk of reflux, without significantly crossing the blood-brain barrier. As a result, it has a lower incidence of central nervous system side effects, such as drowsiness or involuntary muscle movements, which are more commonly associated with other prokinetics like *metoclopramide*.

*Domperidone* is also widely used to increase milk production in lactating women, as it raises **serum prolactin** levels, although this use is off-label in many countries. The drug is available in tablet form, as well as in suspensions for those who have difficulty swallowing pills.

Despite its effectiveness, the use of domperidone has been the subject of safety concerns, particularly regarding its potential effects on the heart. It has been associated with an increased risk of cardiac **arrhythmias** and sudden cardiac death, especially in patients with pre-existing heart conditions or those taking other medications that interact to increase its levels in the blood. Consequently, its use is restricted in some countries and recommended only when the benefits outweigh the potential risks.

Patients prescribed domperidone should be closely monitored for any signs of adverse effects, especially cardiac symptoms. It is critical for healthcare providers to conduct a thorough medical assessment before prescribing domperidone, considering the patient's overall health, existing medical conditions, and concurrent medication use to ensure its safe and effective use.

## <u>Pros</u>

1. **Effective Antiemetic:** *Domperidone* is highly effective at controlling symptoms of nausea and vomiting by blocking *dopamine receptors* in the gut.

2. **Gastrointestinal Motility Improvement:** It enhances gastric emptying and *motility*, making it beneficial for patients with *gastroparesis* and similar gastrointestinal motility disorders.

3. **Low CNS Side Effects:** Because it minimally crosses the blood-brain barrier, domperidone has a lower risk of central nervous system side effects, such as *extrapyramidal symptoms,*

compared to other prokinetic agents like *metoclopramide.*

4. **Lactation Support:** Domperidone can increase *prolactin* levels, which may help in increasing milk supply for lactating mothers, although this use is off-label and requires careful consideration.

# <u>Cons</u>

1. **Cardiac Risk:** *Domperidone* has been associated with an increased risk of serious cardiac side effects, including *QT interval prolongation* and *arrhythmias,* particularly at high doses or in susceptible individuals.

2. **Limited Availability in Some Countries:** Due to concerns about cardiac side effects, its availability is restricted in some countries, including the United States, where it is not FDA approved for any condition.

3. **Potential for Drug Interactions:** Domperidone can interact with other medications, potentially increasing the risk of cardiac side effects or affecting the efficacy of other treatments.

4. **Off-label Use for Lactation:** The use of domperidone to enhance lactation is off-label and not approved in many countries, necessitating

careful consideration and monitoring due to potential risks.

The decision to use *domperidone* involves weighing its benefits in improving gastrointestinal symptoms and aiding lactation against the potential risks, especially cardiac. It requires careful patient selection, adherence to recommended dosages, and monitoring, preferably under the guidance of a healthcare professional.

## Prucalopride Succinate: *Prucalopride Succinate* is a selective *serotonin type 4 (5-HT4) receptor agonist* used primarily in the treatment of *chronic idiopathic constipation (CIC)* in adults. Unlike traditional laxatives that work by increasing the water content in the stool to stimulate bowel movements, prucalopride operates by enhancing the motility of the *gastrointestinal tract*. It stimulates the *serotonin receptors* in the gut, which activates the **peristaltic reflex**, increasing **colonic motility** and facilitating stool passage.

Approved in many countries under the brand name *Motegrity*, prucalopride has shown effectiveness in improving bowel movement frequency, stool consistency, and reducing symptoms associated with constipation, such as straining, bloating, and abdominal discomfort. Its mode of action targets the underlying motor dysfunction in the gastrointestinal system that contributes to *CIC*, making it a valuable option for patients who have not responded adequately to conventional laxatives.

**Prucalopride** is well-tolerated by most patients, with the most common side effects being headache, gastrointestinal disturbances (such as nausea and diarrhea), and abdominal pain. These side effects are generally mild to moderate in intensity and tend to decrease with continued use.

The introduction of prucalopride has been a significant advancement in the management of chronic constipation, offering a mechanism-based treatment option. However, as with any medication, it is important for patients to use prucalopride under the supervision of a healthcare provider to ensure it is appropriate for their specific condition and to monitor for any potential side effects or interactions with other medications. Prucalopride represents a key development in addressing the unmet needs of patients with *CIC*, providing a targeted approach to improving *gastrointestinal motility* and enhancing quality of life.

## Pros

1. **Effective in Treating CIC:** *Prucalopride* has been shown to effectively increase bowel movement frequency and improve stool

consistency, making it a valuable option for patients with CIC.

2. **Targeted Action:** By selectively stimulating $5-HT4$ *receptors*, prucalopride directly targets the underlying cause of constipation without the broad systemic effects associated with non-selective stimulants.

3. **Well-Tolerated:** Generally, prucalopride is well-tolerated by most patients, with a side effect profile that is manageable and less severe than some other treatments for constipation.

4. **Improves Quality of Life:** By alleviating the symptoms of CIC, prucalopride can significantly improve patients' quality of life, including physical and emotional well-being.

## Cons

1. **Gastrointestinal Side Effects:** The most common side effects include headache, gastrointestinal disturbances such as nausea, diarrhea, and abdominal pain, which, while generally mild, can be bothersome to some patients.

2. **Not Suitable for All Patients:** *Prucalopride* should be used with caution in patients with

significant renal impairment and is not recommended for individuals with intestinal perforation or obstruction.

3. **Potential for Drug Interactions:** Although relatively safe, prucalopride may interact with other medications, necessitating careful review of patient medication regimens to avoid adverse interactions.

4. **Cost and Accessibility:** Depending on the healthcare system and insurance coverage, the cost of prucalopride may be a barrier for some patients, and its availability may vary by location.

In summary, *prucalopride succinate* offers an effective and targeted approach to treating *CIC*, with a generally favorable safety profile. However, its use should be individualized based on patient-specific factors, including comorbidities and concomitant medications, to optimize outcomes and minimize adverse effects.

# Mosapride Citrate: *Mosapride Citrate* is a

prokinetic agent that facilitates *gastrointestinal motility*, primarily used in the treatment of various gastrointestinal disorders, such as *gastroesophageal reflux disease (GERD)*, **chronic Gastritis**, and functional *dyspepsia*. It belongs to the class of drugs known as *serotonin (5–HT4) receptor agonists*, which work by stimulating the release of *acetylcholine* in the **enteric nervous system**. This action enhances *gastrointestinal peristalsis*, accelerates gastric emptying, and improves lower esophageal sphincter function, thereby aiding in the digestion and passage of food through the *GI tract*.

Unlike some other *prokinetics*, Mosapride is noted for its selective action on *serotonin receptors*, which tends to minimize the risk of central nervous system side effects, such as anxiety or depression, commonly associated with drugs that cross the blood-brain barrier. However, Mosapride's effectiveness and side effect profile can vary among individuals, and it is generally well tolerated with the most common side effects being mild, such as abdominal pain, diarrhea, and dry mouth.

*Mosapride* is available in several countries, particularly in Asia. In countries where it is prescribed, it offers an important therapeutic option for patients suffering from *motility* disorders, providing relief from symptoms and improving quality of life. Despite its benefits in enhancing *GI motility*, the use of Mosapride, like all medications, requires careful consideration of the potential benefits and risks, patient-specific factors, and the presence of any contraindications. Patients under Mosapride therapy should be monitored for efficacy and adverse effects, ensuring optimal management of their gastrointestinal conditions.

# Pros

1. **Enhanced Gastrointestinal Motility:** Mosapride facilitates gastric emptying and improves intestinal motility, which can significantly alleviate symptoms of *dyspepsia* and *GERD*, such as bloating, nausea, and heartburn.

2. **Selective Action:** By selectively targeting *serotonin receptors* involved in gastrointestinal movement, mosapride promotes motility without the broader side effects seen with less selective agents.

3. **Low Risk of Central Nervous System Side Effects:** Unlike other prokinetic agents that can cross the blood-brain barrier and cause central nervous system side effects, mosapride has a lower risk due to its limited ability to cross the barrier.

4. **Useful in Chronic Treatment:** Its efficacy and safety profile make mosapride suitable for long-term management of chronic gastrointestinal disorders.

# Cons

1. **Limited Availability:** *Mosapride* is not approved for use in some countries, including the United

States, limiting its availability to patients in regions where it is not marketed.

2. **Potential for Drug Interactions:** As with many medications, mosapride can interact with other drugs, particularly those metabolized by the *cytochrome P450 enzyme system*, which could alter drug levels and effects.

3. **Gastrointestinal Side Effects:** Though generally well-tolerated, mosapride can cause gastrointestinal side effects, including diarrhea and abdominal pain, in some patients.

4. **Limited Efficacy in Severe Cases:** While effective for mild to moderate symptoms, mosapride may not be sufficient for severe cases of *gastrointestinal motility* disorders or for patients who do not respond to conventional treatment.

*Mosapride Citrate* offers a beneficial option for improving *gastrointestinal motility* with a relatively favorable safety profile. However, its use should be carefully considered based on the individual patient's condition, potential drug interactions, and availability in their region. Healthcare providers must balance these factors to determine the most appropriate treatment strategy

# Alginates
## Gaviscon Dual Action, Peptac

*Alginates* are naturally occurring *polysaccharides* extracted from brown seaweed, widely utilized in various industries, including food, pharmaceutical, and biomedical, due to their unique properties of gel formation, viscosity, and biocompatibility. In the context of healthcare and medicine, alginates play a significant role, especially in the treatment of *gastroesophageal reflux disease (GERD)* and wound healing.

In the treatment of *GERD*, alginates work by forming a gel-like barrier on top of the stomach contents. This barrier prevents the reflux of acidic and non-acidic stomach contents into the *esophagus*, thus providing relief from the symptoms of heartburn and acid indigestion. When alginates come into contact with *gastric acid*, they undergo a rapid transformation into a viscous gel due to the exchange of *sodium ions* in the alginate with *calcium ions* in the stomach. This gel floats on the surface of the gastric contents, effectively acting as a physical barrier that reduces the risk of acid reflux.

Furthermore, alginates are employed in wound care due to their ability to absorb, exude and maintain a moist environment, which is conducive to healing. They can be formulated into dressings that promote wound healing processes, such as *granulation* and *epithelialization*, and are particularly useful for managing exuding wounds, burns, and ulcers. Alginates' biocompatibility and ease of removal with minimal discomfort make them an ideal choice for wound management, leveraging their natural properties to facilitate healing and improve patient outcomes.

# Alginate Medicines

A couple recognized brand names classified as Alginates available for purchase. Availability might vary based on your geographical location.

## Gaviscon Dual Action: *Gaviscon Dual Action*, almost identically listed under Antacids earlier, is the 2nd mention of the Gaviscon brand. Active ingredients in Gaviscon Dual add a *Sodium Alginate*, along with its *Aluminum Hydroxide*, and *Magnesium Carbonate.* All three of these ingredients work together to provide relief from the symptoms of acid reflux and heartburn by neutralizing stomach acid while ALSO forming a protective barrier to prevent acid from re-entering the *esophagus*.

Gaviscon is available in various forms, including tablets and liquid. Always refer to the specific product label for the most accurate information on active compounds.

# Peptac: *Peptac* is an over-the-counter medication used to relieve symptoms of heartburn and indigestion. It contains three active ingredients that work together to neutralize stomach acid: ***Sodium Alginate***, ***Sodium Bicarbonate***, and ***Calcium Carbonate***. Additional antacid components that help to neutralize stomach acid and relieve symptoms of indigestion and heartburn.

*Peptac* is available in liquid form and is designed to provide symptomatic relief from *(GERD)*, heartburn, and indigestion. The combination of these compounds offers effective relief by both neutralizing stomach acid and forming a barrier to prevent acid reflux. Always consult the product packaging or leaflet for a complete list of ingredients and to ensure it is suitable for your specific health needs, especially if you have allergies or other medical conditions.

# Alginate Medicines
## Compounds Used – Pros & Cons

* Sodium Alginate (Aluminum Hydroxide, Magnesium Carbonate, Sodium Bicarbonate, Calcium Carbonate)

** **Note**: Apart from Sodium Alginate mentioned immediately below, components such as Aluminum Hydroxide, Magnesium Carbonate, Sodium Bicarbonate, and Calcium Carbonate have previously been identified as ingredients common in numerous antacid formulas. Medications containing alginate add an extra layer of protection to these neutralizing agents present in antacids. These are re-listed here for your convenience.*

**Sodium Alginate:** *Sodium Alginate* is a natural *polysaccharide* derived from brown seaweed, widely recognized for its unique properties and versatility in various industries, including pharmaceuticals, food, and textile. In the medical field, *sodium alginate* plays a crucial role, particularly in the treatment of *gastroesophageal reflux disease (GERD)* and heartburn. It operates by reacting with *gastric acid* to form a viscous gel or raft that floats on the stomach contents, acting as a physical barrier that prevents the reflux of stomach acid back into the *esophagus*. This mechanism effectively reduces the symptoms of heartburn and discomfort associated with acid reflux.

## Pros

1. **Effective Symptom Relief:** *Sodium alginate* quickly forms a protective barrier in the stomach, offering rapid relief from the discomfort of heartburn and acid reflux.

2. **Natural Origin:** Being derived from seaweed, it is a natural remedy, which can be appealing to those seeking alternatives to *synthetic medications*.

3. **Safe for Long-Term Use:** It is generally considered safe for extended periods, with fewer side effects compared to long-term use of traditional acid-suppressing medications like *proton pump inhibitors (PPIs)* and *H2 blockers*.

4. **Minimal Systemic Absorption:** Sodium alginate works locally in the stomach without being significantly absorbed into the bloodstream, minimizing systemic side effects.

## Cons

1. **Limited Effectiveness for Severe GERD:** While effective for mild to moderate symptoms of acid

reflux, it may not be sufficient for severe *GERD* cases or for those with significant esophageal damage.

2. **Potential for Drug Interactions:** It can bind to certain medications in the stomach, potentially affecting their absorption and efficacy.

3. **Gastrointestinal Side Effects:** Some users may experience gastrointestinal side effects such as bloating or constipation due to the gel-like substance formed by alginate.

4. **Allergic Reactions:** Although rare, allergic reactions to *sodium alginate* can occur, especially in individuals sensitive to seaweed or other components.

In summary, *sodium alginate* is a valuable option for managing heartburn and *GERD* symptoms, offering a natural and effective remedy with minimal systemic effects. However, its suitability may vary based on the severity of the condition, potential interactions with other medications, and individual patient sensitivities. Always consult with a healthcare provider to determine the most appropriate treatment for your specific needs.

# **Aluminum Hydroxide:** *Aluminum hydroxide* is an antacid medication commonly used to treat symptoms of excess stomach acid, such as heartburn, acid indigestion, and upset stomach. It works by neutralizing stomach acid, thereby providing relief from discomfort. Beyond its antacid properties, *aluminum hydroxide* is also used to reduce phosphate levels in people with certain kidney conditions, helping to prevent the formation of kidney stones by binding phosphate in the intestines.

Available in various forms, including tablets, capsules, and liquid suspensions, aluminum hydroxide is accessible and easy to use. However, it's important for users to follow dosing instructions carefully to avoid side effects such as constipation, which is a common issue with aluminum-containing antacids. In some cases, long-term use can lead to aluminum accumulation, particularly in individuals with kidney problems, leading to potential health risks. Therefore, while *aluminum hydroxide* is effective for temporary relief of stomach acid-related symptoms, it should be used judiciously and under the guidance of a healthcare professional, especially for individuals with pre-existing health conditions.

*Aluminum hydroxide* is commonly used in medicine as an antacid and *phosphate binder*, offering relief from symptoms of increased stomach acidity such as heartburn, upset stomach, and indigestion. It also helps reduce phosphate levels in people with certain kidney conditions.

## Pros

1. **Effective Antacid:** *Aluminum hydroxide* effectively neutralizes stomach acid, providing quick relief from acid-related symptoms.

2. **Phosphate Binder:** It is beneficial for patients with chronic kidney disease by reducing phosphate absorption in the intestines, thus helping manage *serum phosphate levels.*

3. **Safety Profile:** Generally considered safe for short-term use in appropriate doses, with minimal systemic absorption.

4. **Versatile Use:** Available in various forms, such as tablets, capsules, and liquid, making it accessible for different patient needs and preferences.

## Cons

1. **Constipation:** One of the most common side effects is constipation, which can be

uncomfortable and require management with diet or medication.

2. **Potential for Aluminum Toxicity:** With long-term use, especially in patients with renal impairment, there's a risk of aluminum accumulation leading to toxicity, affecting the central nervous system and bones.

3. **Drug Interactions:** *Aluminum hydroxide* can interfere with the absorption of several medications, including antibiotics and heart medications, potentially reducing their effectiveness.

4. **Nutrient Absorption:** It may also interfere with the absorption of certain nutrients, such as iron, leading to deficiencies if used over a long period.

While aluminum hydroxide can be an effective treatment for managing symptoms of excess stomach acid and controlling phosphate levels in kidney patients, its use should be carefully considered against potential side effects and interactions. It's important for patients to follow medical advice and dosage recommendations to minimize risks.

# Magnesium Hydroxide: *Magnesium*

*hydroxide* is an inorganic compound commonly used as an antacid and a laxative, recognized for its ability to neutralize stomach acid and relieve symptoms of indigestion, heartburn, and sour stomach. It works by reacting with *hydrochloric acid* in the stomach to form *magnesium chloride* and water, thereby reducing acidity and providing symptomatic relief from discomfort caused by excess stomach acid.

As a laxative, *magnesium hydroxide* operates by drawing water into the intestines, which helps to soften the stool and promotes intestinal movements, aiding in the relief of occasional constipation.

Available over the counter in various forms, including liquid suspensions and tablets, magnesium hydroxide is known for its quick onset of action and safety profile when used as directed. However, it's essential for users to adhere to recommended dosages to avoid potential side effects such as diarrhea or *electrolyte imbalances*. Long-term use or overuse should be avoided unless supervised by a healthcare provider, as it may lead to dependency for bowel function or affect the balance of minerals in the body.

# **<u>Pros</u>**

1. **Effective Antacid:** *Magnesium hydroxide* quickly neutralizes stomach acid, providing relief from indigestion, heartburn, and acid reflux. This can improve quality of life for those suffering from these conditions.

2. **Gentle Laxative:** As a laxative, it works by drawing water into the intestines, which helps soften the stool and promotes bowel movements. This mechanism is gentle and considered safe for occasional use.

3. **Minimal Systemic Absorption:** It has minimal systemic absorption, which makes it a safer option compared to other medications that are absorbed into the bloodstream and may have widespread effects.

4. **Availability:** It is readily available over the counter in various forms, making it easily accessible for those in need of quick relief.

5. **Safe for Kidneys:** In patients with normal kidney function, it can be safer than other antacids that contain aluminum or calcium, which can cause problems in individuals with renal issues.

## <u>Cons</u>

1. **Hypermagnesemia Risk:** In patients with renal impairment, there's a risk of *hypermagnesemia* (high magnesium levels in the blood) due to decreased ability to excrete magnesium, which can lead to serious side effects.

2. **Diarrhea:** Overuse as a laxative can lead to diarrhea, which may result in dehydration and *electrolyte imbalances* if not properly managed.

3. **Interactions with Medications:** Magnesium hydroxide can interfere with the absorption of certain medications, including some antibiotics and bisphosphonates, reducing their effectiveness.

4. **Dependency:** With prolonged use as a laxative, there's a risk of becoming dependent on it for bowel movements, potentially leading to a cycle where natural bowel function is diminished.

5. **Limited Long-Term Use:** Due to potential side effects and interactions, magnesium hydroxide is not recommended for long-term use without medical supervision.

In summary, *magnesium hydroxide* offers significant benefits for treating acid-related disorders and constipation with minimal side effects when used appropriately. However, its cons highlight the importance of careful and informed use, especially in individuals with underlying health conditions or those taking other medications.

## Sodium Bicarbonate: *Sodium*

*Bicarbonate* commonly known as baking soda, is a versatile compound with a wide range of uses, including medical applications. Chemically, it is represented as $NaHCO_3$ and is a white, crystalline powder that is slightly alkaline in taste. In the medical field, *sodium bicarbonate* is primarily used as an antacid to treat conditions like heartburn, acid indigestion, and upset stomach by neutralizing stomach acid, providing quick relief from discomfort.

Beyond its antacid properties, *sodium bicarbonate* is also utilized in emergency medicine as an intravenous infusion to correct acidosis in patients with severe metabolic acidosis, a condition where the body produces excessive acid or the kidneys are not removing enough acid from the body.

Additionally, it serves a role in the treatment of certain drug intoxications, including tricyclic antidepressant overdose, by helping to normalize the body's pH balance. Despite its benefits, careful administration is necessary to avoid side effects, such as metabolic alkalosis, especially in patients with underlying health conditions.

Sodium bicarbonate, widely known as baking soda, is used medically for its antacid properties and ability to manage acid-base imbalances. Here are the pros and cons of its medical use:

## <u>Pros</u>

1. **Rapid Acid Neutralization:** *Sodium bicarbonate* effectively neutralizes stomach acid, providing quick relief from conditions like heartburn, acid indigestion, and upset stomach.

2. **Treatment of Acidosis:** It is used in emergency medicine to correct metabolic acidosis, a condition where the body has too much acid, helping to restore the body's pH balance.

3. **Versatile Medical Uses:** Beyond treating acid-related conditions, it's used in the management of certain drug overdoses and poisoning by helping to increase the pH of urine, which facilitates the excretion of certain substances.

4. **Availability:** It is readily available, inexpensive, and can be administered orally or intravenously,

making it accessible for a variety of medical situations.

## Cons

1. **Electrolyte Imbalance:** With excessive use, *sodium bicarbonate* can lead to *electrolyte imbalances*, particularly *hypernatremia* (high sodium levels) and hypokalemia (low potassium levels).

2. **Alkalosis Risk:** Overuse or incorrect administration can result in *metabolic alkalosis*, where the body's pH becomes too high, leading to muscle twitching, hand tremors, and other symptoms.

3. **Gastrointestinal Side Effects:** Oral administration can cause gastrointestinal issues like bloating and gas due to the release of carbon dioxide gas when it neutralizes stomach acid.

4. **Interactions with Medications:** It can interact with various medications, altering their absorption and effectiveness, which requires careful management in patients on multiple medications.

In medical practice, the use of *sodium bicarbonate* must be carefully balanced, considering the patient's overall health, existing conditions, and potential risks associated with its use.

## Calcium Carbonate: *Calcium carbonate* is a widely prevalent compound found naturally in rocks, pearls, and the shells of marine organisms. Its chemical formula is $CaCO_3$, embodying a combination of calcium, carbon, and oxygen. This compound is the principal component of limestone, chalk, and marble, three of the most common forms of *calcium carbonate* found in nature. Due to its vast availability and versatile properties, calcium carbonate has a broad range of applications both industrially and medically.

In the medical field, calcium carbonate is extensively used as a calcium supplement and antacid. As a supplement, it helps prevent and treat calcium deficiencies and conditions related to low bone density, such as *osteoporosis*. Its antacid properties offer quick relief from symptoms of heartburn, acid indigestion, and upset stomach by neutralizing stomach acid.

Furthermore, calcium carbonate is favored for its high calcium content and cost-effectiveness, making it a popular choice among calcium supplements. However, its effectiveness as a calcium source is dependent on stomach acid for absorption, making it less suitable for individuals with reduced stomach acid levels.

Interestingly, besides its medical uses, calcium carbonate is also a critical ingredient in the manufacture of cement and lime, and as a filler and coating agent in the production of paper, plastics, and paint, showcasing its versatility across various industries.

## **Pros**

1. **Effective Antacid:** It quickly neutralizes stomach acid, providing relief from heartburn, acid indigestion, and an upset stomach.

2. **Calcium Supplementation:** As a source of calcium, it helps in the prevention and treatment of *osteoporosis* by supporting bone health and maintenance.

3. **Cost-Effective:** Compared to other calcium supplements, calcium carbonate is relatively inexpensive and widely available.

4. **Versatile Forms:** Available in various forms (tablets, capsules, chewables, liquids), making it accessible for different age groups and preferences.

## **Cons**

1. **Absorption Issues:** *Calcium carbonate* requires stomach acid for best absorption, so it may be

less effective when taken on an empty stomach or for individuals with low stomach acid.

2. **Gastrointestinal Side Effects:** Can cause gas, bloating, and constipation in some individuals, especially when taken in high doses.

3. **Risk of Overuse:** Excessive consumption can lead to *hypercalcemia* (high calcium levels in the blood), which can affect kidney function and lead to kidney stones.

4. **Interactions:** It can interfere with the absorption of other medications, such as *bisphosphonates* (used to treat *osteoporosis*) and some antibiotics, reducing their effectiveness.

In medical use, the choice to use *calcium carbonate* should consider these pros and cons, balancing its benefits against potential side effects or interactions with other medications. It's important for individuals to consult healthcare professionals before starting any new supplement, especially if they have underlying health conditions or are taking other medications.

# Coating agents
## Pepto-Bismol, Kaopectate

*Coating agents* are used for managing heartburn function by forming a protective barrier on the stomach lining and *esophagus*, shielding them from the corrosive effects of gastric acid. These agents are integral to the treatment of conditions such as *gastroesophageal reflux disease (GERD)* and heartburn, offering symptomatic relief by directly targeting the discomfort caused by acid reflux.

The mechanism of action for these coating agents involves their physical properties rather than altering the pH of the stomach acid or reducing its production. When ingested, these substances can quickly interact with the gastric contents to form a viscous, gel-like layer. This gel acts as a mechanical barrier that floats on top of the stomach contents, preventing acid from rising into the *esophagus* and causing the burning sensation associated with heartburn.

Some *coating agents* contain *alginates*, which are particularly effective in this role. Upon contact with *gastric acid*, alginates undergo a reaction that allows them to form a raft-like structure. This structure is less dense than the stomach fluids, enabling it to remain on the surface of the gastric contents and effectively block the reflux of acid and bile into the *esophagus*.

In addition to providing immediate relief from heartburn symptoms, these coating agents can also protect the damaged mucosal lining of the *esophagus* and stomach, allowing it time to heal. They are often used as an over-the-counter remedy for mild symptoms of acid reflux and can be a part of a broader treatment regimen for more severe forms of *GERD*, often in combination with acid suppressants like *proton pump inhibitors* or *H2 receptor antagonists* for comprehensive management of the condition.

## Coating Agent Medicines

Here are a couple well-known brand name Coating Agents available for purchase depending on your regional area.

**Pepto-Bismol:** *Pepto–Bismol* is a well-known over-the-counter medication used to treat temporary discomforts of the stomach and *gastrointestinal tract*, such as indigestion, nausea, heartburn, upset stomach, and diarrhea. The primary active ingredient in Pepto-Bismol is **Bismuth Subsalicylate**. This compound has *antacid* and mild antibacterial properties. It works by coating the stomach lining, reducing inflammation and irritation, and inhibiting the growth of bacteria that can cause diarrhea and other gastrointestinal symptoms.

In addition to *bismuth subsalicylate*, Pepto-Bismol may contain several inactive ingredients, which can vary depending on the specific product form (liquid, chewable tablets, caplets).

It's important to note that Pepto-Bismol should be used according to package instructions or a healthcare provider's guidance. Due to its **salicylate content**, it should not be used by children or teenagers with flu symptoms or chickenpox due to the risk of **Reye's syndrome**, a rare but serious condition. Always check the label for the complete list of ingredients and any specific warnings or instructions

# Kaopectate: *Kaopectate* is an over-the-counter medication traditionally used to treat mild diarrhea, upset stomach, and indigestion. Almost identical to Pepto-Bismol in that it utilizes the same medical ingredient **Bismuth Subsalicylate**. This compound acts as an anti-inflammatory, *antacid*, and mild antibiotic. It works by coating the stomach lining, reducing the inflammation and irritation caused by stomach acids, and can inhibit the growth of bacteria that cause diarrhea and other gastrointestinal symptoms.

In addition to *bismuth subsalicylate*, Kaopectate may contain inactive ingredients that vary depending on the product form (liquid, caplets). These can include flavoring agents, coloring agents, and other compounds to enhance the product's stability and usability.

It's important to note that, due to its content of bismuth subsalicylate, Kaopectate should not be used by children or teenagers with flu symptoms or chickenpox due to the risk of **Reye's syndrome**, a rare but serious condition.

Always follow the product's instructions for use and consult with a healthcare provider if you have any questions or concerns about its use, especially in children or if you are pregnant or breastfeeding.

# Coating Agent Medicines
## Compounds Used – Pros & Cons

Bismuth Subsalicylate

## **Bismuth Subsalicylate:** *Bismuth*

*Subsalicylate* is a widely used over-the-counter medication, most commonly recognized as the active ingredient in products like Pepto-Bismol and Kaopectate. It serves multiple roles in managing gastrointestinal disorders, functioning as an anti-inflammatory, *antacid*, and mild antibiotic. This versatile compound is effective in treating symptoms such as nausea, heartburn, indigestion, upset stomach, and diarrhea.

Its mechanism of action includes coating the stomach lining, thereby protecting it from irritants and acid, and its **antimicrobial properties** can reduce harmful bacteria in the *gastrointestinal tract*, including *Helicobacter pylori*, which is often implicated in ulcers and *gastritis*.

Additionally, *bismuth subsalicylate* has the unique side effect of temporarily darkening the user's stool and tongue, a harmless but notable reaction. While it offers significant relief for various digestive symptoms, its use is cautioned against in children and teenagers recovering from viral infections due to the risk of *Reye's syndrome*, a rare but serious condition.

# <u>Pros</u>

1. **Broad Symptom Relief:** *Bismuth subsalicylate* effectively relieves a wide range of gastrointestinal symptoms, making it a versatile option for symptomatic treatment.

2. **Antimicrobial Effects:** It possesses mild *antimicrobial properties* that can reduce the number of bacteria in the gut, including *Helicobacter pylori*, which is often associated with ulcers and *gastritis*.

3. **Protective Coating Action:** The medication forms a protective barrier over the stomach lining and ulcers, shielding them from stomach acid and allowing them to heal.

4. **Anti-Inflammatory Properties:** Bismuth subsalicylate can help reduce inflammation in the stomach and intestines, contributing to symptom relief.

# <u>Cons</u>

1. **Reye's Syndrome Risk:** It should not be used in children or teenagers recovering from viral infections, especially influenza or chickenpox, due to the risk of *Reye's syndrome*, a rare but serious condition.

2. **Black Stool and Tongue:** A harmless but potentially alarming side effect is the temporary darkening of the stool and tongue caused by the bismuth component.

3. **Drug Interactions:** Bismuth subsalicylate can interact with other medications, including *tetracycline antibiotics* and *anticoagulants* like warfarin, potentially affecting their efficacy.

4. **Allergic Reactions:** Though rare, some individuals may experience allergic reactions to salicylates, including bismuth subsalicylate.

5. **Chronic Use Issues:** Prolonged use can lead to bismuth toxicity, characterized by neurological symptoms such as confusion and coordination problems, though this is extremely rare.

In summary, *bismuth subsalicylate* is a useful medication for temporary relief from a variety of gastrointestinal symptoms. However, its use should be carefully considered, especially in children, teenagers, and individuals taking certain other medications. Always consult a healthcare provider for advice tailored to your specific health situation.

# TWELVE
## Generic Medicines vs. Name Brand

Many of the largest drugstore chains have developed their own generic brand names for a wide range of products, from over-the-counter medications to health and wellness items. These private label brands offer consumers more affordable alternatives to name-brand products without compromising on quality.

Understanding the labeling of store-branded generic medications is absolutely essential. First, these medicines will typically list the store's generic name, but next will clearly indicate the active ingredients used. For instance, Walmart's "Equate" brand covers a wide range of medical compounds, but uses the same active ingredients as more expensive name brands.

Brand name examples such as: Prilosec, Nexium, Tagamet, Pepcid, Rolaids, and Pepto Bismol each feature unique ingredients. However in the following example; Walmart's Equate brand covers all of them under their generic name Equate, but focusing on the active compounds used.

# Examples of 'Equate' (Walmart Brand) Acid Reflux products

## <u>Typically will be labeled:</u>

EQUATE → *Omeprazole* (Brand Name, **Prilosec**)

EQUATE → *Lansoprazole* (Brand Name, **Nexium**)

EQUATE → *Cimetidine* (Brand Name, **Tagamet**)

EQUATE → *Famotidine* (Brand Name, **Pepcid**)

EQUATE → *Bismuth Subsalicylate*
       (Brand Name, **Pepto Bismol**)

~~~~~~~~~~~~~~~~~~~~~~~~~~~~~~~~~~~~~

On Occasion the label will list the type of medicine first, then the generic private label, and always the active ingredient used such as:

Antacid Tablets - EQUATE → *Calcium Carbonate* (Equivalent brand name, **Tums**)

~~~~~~~~~~~~~~~~~~~~~~~~~~~~~~~~~~~~~

This approach is consistent across major drugstore chains, highlighting a common strategy of offering generic alternatives to name-brand medications focusing on the active ingredients.

Several mega pharmacy chains that have their own generic brand names, along with examples of their private labels:

# Walmart

- Generic Brand: *Equate*

Offers a comprehensive range of health-related products, including pharmacy, nutritional supplements, and personal care items.

# Walgreens

- Generic Brand: *Walgreens Brand*
- Offers a wide array of health products, including over-the-counter medications, first aid supplies, and personal care items.

# CVS Pharmacy

- Generic Brand: *CVS Health*
- Features an extensive selection of health products, including pharmacy items, health supplements, and personal care products.

# Rite Aid

- Generic Brand: *Rite Aid Pharmacy*
- Provides a variety of health and wellness products, including over-the-counter

medications, vitamins, and personal care items.

# Target

- Generic Brand: ***Up&Up***
- Features a broad selection of health and wellness products, including over-the-counter medications, first aid, and beauty products.

# Costco

- Generic Brand: ***Kirkland Signature***
- Known for its high-quality, value-priced health products, including over-the-counter medications, vitamins, and supplements.

# Kroger

- Generic Brand: ***Kroger Brand***
- Provides a variety of pharmacy and health products, including over-the-counter medications and nutritional supplements.

# Albertsons (including Safeway, Vons, and others)

- Generic Brand: ***Signature Care***

- Offers a range of health products, including over-the-counter medications, first aid supplies, and personal care items.

## Publix

- Generic Brand: **Publix Brand**
- Features a selection of health and wellness products, including pharmacy items, vitamins, and personal care products.

## H-E-B

- Generic Brand: ***H-E-B Brand***
- Offers health products, including over-the-counter medications, first aid supplies, and personal care items.

These generic brands have become popular for their quality and affordability, allowing consumers to save money without sacrificing effectiveness. Each of these chains has successfully leveraged their brand to build trust and loyalty among their customer base, making their generic products a go-to choice for many shoppers.

# Features to Consider

When considering medication options, patients and healthcare providers often weigh the merits of generic versus brand-name medicines. This comparison looks at a range of factors, including efficacy (effectiveness), cost, availability, regulatory standards, patient perception, and pharmaceutical innovation.

## Efficacy and Quality

Generic medicines contain the same active ingredients as their brand-name counterparts and are required by regulatory agencies, such as the *FDA* in the United States, to demonstrate *bioequivalence*. This means that generics must perform similarly in the body to the brand-name original. Studies consistently support the conclusion that generics are as effective and safe as brand-name drugs. However, despite this equivalence, some patients and healthcare professionals report perceived differences in effectiveness or side effects, possibly due to variances in inactive ingredients or psychological factors.

## Cost and Accessibility

The most apparent advantage of generic medicines is their lower cost, which can be 80-85% less than brand-name drugs. This price difference makes generics a pivotal option for improving healthcare affordability and access. The lower cost of generics is attributed to the competition among manufacturers once patent protections expire for the brand-name drug, eliminating the need for generics to recoup the original drug's research, development, and marketing expenses.

## Regulatory Standards

Both generic and brand-name drugs are subject to stringent regulatory standards for approval, manufacturing, and quality control. However, brand-name drugs undergo extensive clinical trials to demonstrate safety and efficacy before hitting the market, a process that can take many years and significant investment. In contrast, generic manufacturers need only prove *bioequivalence* to existing medications, streamlining their path to market.

## Patient Perception and Trust

Patient perception can significantly influence medication effectiveness, known as the ***placebo effect***. Some patients report a preference for brand-name medications, believing them to be more effective or safer than generics. This perception can impact compliance and satisfaction with treatment, despite evidence supporting generic efficacy. Educational efforts by healthcare providers are crucial in building trust and understanding regarding generic medications.

## Pharmaceutical Innovation

The development of brand-name drugs plays a crucial role in advancing medical science and treatment options. The high cost of these drugs partially reflects the significant investment in research and development, including the cost of drugs that fail to reach the market. Critics of generic dominance argue that it could reduce the financial incentives for such innovation. Conversely, the availability of generics after patent expiration ensures that once novel treatments become accessible to a broader patient base, supporting public health.

## Environmental and Ethical Considerations

Generic manufacturing might have a less pronounced environmental impact than brand-name drug production, given the reduced need for extensive clinical trials and associated activities. However, ethical considerations, such as patent disputes, marketing practices, and access to life-saving medications in low-income countries, are complex issues affecting both sectors.

## Global Market Dynamics

The generic drug market has significantly expanded access to medications worldwide, particularly in developing countries where cost barriers limit access to brand-name drugs. This global availability has improved treatment outcomes for millions but also introduced challenges, such as quality control and counterfeit drugs, which require ongoing vigilance from international regulatory bodies.

## Summary

Generic and name-brand medications serve essential roles within healthcare, offering patients options for treatment based on efficacy, cost, and availability. Generics, identical in active ingredients and dosage to their brand-name counterparts, are rigorously tested to ensure *bioequivalence*, guaranteeing similar therapeutic outcomes.

Their primary advantage lies in affordability, typically costing 80-85% less than brand-name drugs, which significantly enhances access to vital medications for broader populations. The lower cost stems from generics not having to recoup the original drug's extensive research, development, and marketing expenses.

Conversely, brand-name medications are the pioneers of pharmaceutical innovation, introducing new treatments to the market after undergoing rigorous clinical trials to prove safety and effectiveness. While they command higher prices, reflecting the investment in their development, they also build patient trust and brand loyalty.

Despite their differences, both generic and brand-name drugs adhere to strict regulatory standards ensuring safety and effectiveness. Patient perceptions vary, with some showing preference for brand names due to perceived efficacy or concerns about generics' quality. Ultimately, the choice between generic and brand-name medications should consider individual patient needs, healthcare provider recommendations, and the specific clinical scenario, aiming to balance quality care with cost-effectiveness and accessibility.

## Crucial Final Point ♡

Understanding the similarities and differences between generic store-branded medications and name brand labels is extremely important. Equally as important is being able to identify, recognize and understand these generic medications for purchase next time you're in the store.

I strongly suggest bringing this book along as your reference guide during your next visit to any pharmacy, especially when searching for medications to treat heartburn and acid reflux. Armed with the knowledge this book provides, you are now equipped to make informed and confident decisions regarding your health care.

This book also includes an extensive Glossary of Terms with page number reference. Simply look up the medical compound in the glossary, and it will indicate the page number within this book that each ingredient has been previously explained in comprehensive detail.

# THIRTEEN
## DOSAGE - Factors to Evaluate

Dosage variations among individuals for a given medication can be attributed to several key factors, each aiming to optimize therapeutic outcomes while minimizing the risk of side effects. Here are the primary reasons why different dosages may be prescribed:

1.  **Body Weight:** Individual body weight and size are pivotal factors in determining the appropriate dosage of medication for an individual. This is because the *pharmacokinetics* of a drug—how it's absorbed, distributed, metabolized, and excreted—can vary significantly with the body mass and composition of the patient. A primary goal in prescribing medication is to achieve a therapeutic effect while minimizing side effects, and tailoring the dose to the patient's body weight and size is a key strategy in achieving this balance.

    For many medications, dosing guidelines are based on weight, especially in pediatrics, to ensure safety and efficacy. The rationale is straightforward: a larger body may require more of a drug to reach the same concentration in the bloodstream that a smaller body would achieve with a lesser amount. Conversely, a dose that is too high for a smaller individual can lead to increased risk of adverse effects without providing additional therapeutic benefit.

Moreover, body composition, including the ratio of fat to muscle, can influence drug distribution. *Lipophilic (fat-soluble) drugs*, for example, may have a longer duration of action in individuals with higher body fat percentages due to greater storage capacity, necessitating adjustments in dosing or frequency.

In addition to weight and size, other factors like body surface area (BSA) are sometimes considered for more precise dosing of certain drugs, particularly in cancer chemotherapy, where BSA can provide a better approximation of metabolic mass than weight alone.

Ultimately, considering body weight and size in dosing is essential for personalized medicine, ensuring that each patient receives the most effective and safest drug regimen tailored to their individual needs.

2.  **Age:** Considering age when determining medication dosage for adults is crucial, as physiological changes that occur with aging can significantly impact drug *pharmacokinetics* and *pharmacodynamics*. Adults, spanning from young adulthood to advanced age, exhibit a wide range of variations in body composition, organ function, and metabolic rates, all of which are essential factors in medication metabolism and elimination.

    In younger adults, robust metabolic and excretory functions typically allow for standard dosing regimens to be effective and safe. However, as individuals age, there's a gradual decline in organ function, particularly in the liver and kidneys, which play pivotal roles in drug metabolism and clearance. For instance, *hepatic enzyme* activity may decrease, and renal blood flow and *glomerular filtration rate* tend to decline, extending the half-life of many drugs and increasing the potential for drug accumulation and toxicity.

    Moreover, age-related changes in body composition, such as increased body fat and decreased lean body mass and body water, can alter the distribution of water-soluble and fat-soluble drugs, respectively. These changes necessitate adjustments in dosage to avoid adverse effects while maintaining therapeutic efficacy.

Additionally, older adults are more likely to suffer from multiple chronic conditions, leading to *polypharmacy*, which increases the risk of drug-drug interactions and further complicates dosing considerations. Therefore, a careful, individualized approach to medication dosing is essential, often starting with lower doses and adjusting based on response and side effects, to ensure optimal care for adults as they age.

3. **Gender:** Gender can also play a significant role in determining the appropriate dosage of medications for adults due to differences in body composition, hormonal levels, and metabolic processes between males and females. Women often have a higher percentage of body fat and a lower percentage of water than men, which can affect the distribution and elimination of certain drugs. Hormonal fluctuations in women, particularly due to menstrual cycles, pregnancy, or menopause, can also influence drug metabolism and efficacy. Therefore, gender-specific considerations are crucial to tailor medication dosages for optimal efficacy and minimized risk of adverse effects.

4. **Kidney and Liver Function:** Kidney and liver functions are paramount considerations when determining medication dosage for adults, as these organs are central to the metabolism and excretion of drugs. The liver primarily metabolizes drugs, transforming them into more water-soluble compounds for elimination. The kidneys further filter these metabolites out of the bloodstream and excrete them through urine. Any impairment in these organs can significantly impact a drug's *pharmacokinetics*, potentially leading to accumulation and increased risk of toxicity.

   In adults with renal impairment, the decreased filtration rate can prolong the half-life of renally excreted medications, necessitating dosage adjustments or interval extensions to prevent drug accumulation and adverse effects. Drugs or their *metabolites* that are normally excreted by the kidneys can reach toxic levels if not properly dosed according to renal function, measured by *creatinine clearance* or *glomerular filtration rate (GFR)*.

   Similarly, liver disease affects drug metabolism by reducing the organ's capacity to biotransform drugs. This can lead to higher systemic concentrations of medications, requiring dose reductions or alternative therapies to avoid toxicity. The liver's role in producing proteins that bind drugs also changes with disease, affecting drug bioavailability and distribution.

For adults with compromised kidney or liver function, healthcare providers must meticulously adjust dosages, considering the severity of organ impairment, the drug's therapeutic index, and the specific pharmacological properties of the medication. This often involves initiating therapy at lower doses, closely monitoring for efficacy and toxicity, and possibly utilizing drugs with alternative elimination pathways.

Understanding the intricacies of how *renal* and *hepatic functions* influence drug kinetics is crucial for clinicians to optimize therapeutic outcomes while minimizing risks, underscoring the importance of individualized medication management based on the patient's organ function status.

5. **Genetics:** Genetics play a critical role in medication dosing for adults due to variations in genes that encode drug-metabolizing enzymes, transporters, and receptors. These genetic differences can profoundly influence an individual's response to medications, categorizing them as slow, intermediate, fast, or ultra-fast metabolizers. For example, variations in the *CYP450 enzyme family* affect the metabolism of

many drugs, leading to variability in drug efficacy and risk of adverse effects.

Personalized medicine, which includes pharmacogenomic testing, helps tailor medication dosages to an individual's genetic profile, optimizing therapeutic outcomes and minimizing toxicity by predicting metabolic rates and responses to specific medications.

6. **Drug Interactions:** Considering drug interactions is crucial when determining medication dosages for adults. Use of multiple medications can lead to interactions that affect the *pharmacokinetics* or *pharmacodynamics* of one or more of the involved drugs. These interactions may enhance or diminish the efficacy of a medication, potentially leading to adverse effects or therapeutic failure. Adjusting dosages or selecting alternative medications becomes essential to mitigate such risks, emphasizing the importance of a thorough medication review by healthcare professionals to ensure safe and effective treatment regimens.

7. **Tolerance** (or Desensitization): Long-term use Tolerance is a significant factor in adjusting medication dosages for adults, referring to the body's reduced response to a drug after prolonged use. This phenomenon necessitates higher doses

to achieve the same therapeutic effect initially observed. Tolerance can develop due to changes in drug metabolism, receptor sensitivity, or physiological adaptations. It's commonly seen with medications for pain management, anxiety, and sleep disorders.

Recognizing and managing tolerance is crucial to prevent escalation of doses that could lead to dependency, adverse effects, or overdose. Healthcare providers may counteract tolerance by rotating medications, prescribing drug holidays, or employing combination therapies to maintain efficacy while minimizing risks.

8. **Severity of Condition:** The severity of a medical condition is a pivotal factor in determining the appropriate medication dosage for adults. This principle ensures that the therapeutic intervention is adequately potent to manage the condition effectively without causing unnecessary side effects. For serious or acute conditions, higher doses might be necessary to quickly control symptoms and stabilize the patient. Such scenarios demand an aggressive treatment approach to mitigate the risk of complications or progression of the disease. Conversely, in managing chronic or less severe conditions, a more conservative dosage might be preferred to

minimize side effects, especially for long-term treatment strategies.

Adjusting dosages based on the condition's severity also involves a dynamic assessment process. As the patient's condition improves or deteriorates, healthcare providers may need to recalibrate the dosage to adapt to the changing clinical needs. This careful balancing act aims to maintain an optimal therapeutic window, where the benefits of the medication outweigh the risks of adverse reactions.

Moreover, the severity of the condition influences not just the dosage but also the choice of medication. In some cases, a combination of drugs at lower doses may be employed to manage a condition effectively, reducing the risk of side effects associated with higher doses of a single medication. Ultimately, considering the severity of the condition allows for a tailored approach to medication management, ensuring that each patient receives the most appropriate and effective treatment.

9. **Compliance and Lifestyle Factors:**
Compliance and lifestyle factors are critical considerations when determining medication dosages for adults. Adherence to prescribed treatment regimens ensures the effectiveness of

medication, while non-compliance can lead to suboptimal therapeutic outcomes. Lifestyle factors, including diet, exercise, smoking, and alcohol consumption, can also significantly impact medication metabolism and efficacy. For instance, certain foods and beverages may interact with drugs, altering their absorption or effect, while habits like smoking can accelerate the metabolism of some medications, requiring dosage adjustments. Tailoring dosages to accommodate individual lifestyle factors and emphasizing the importance of compliance are essential strategies to optimize treatment effectiveness and patient well-being.

10. **Individual Response:** The concept of individual response is crucial in the realm of pharmacotherapy, especially when determining the appropriate medication dosage for adults. This principle acknowledges that each person's body uniquely processes and responds to medications due to a complex interplay of genetic, physiological, and environmental factors. As such, healthcare providers must consider these individual differences to optimize therapeutic outcomes and minimize the risk of adverse effects.

Genetic makeup is a significant determinant of individual response, influencing drug metabolism rates, efficacy, and the likelihood of side effects. Variations in genes that encode for drug-metabolizing enzymes, drug transporters, and drug targets can significantly affect a patient's response to a given medication. For example, *polymorphisms* in the *cytochrome P450 enzymes* can render some individuals as slow metabolizers, who may experience enhanced drug effects or increased side effects at standard doses, while fast metabolizers may require higher doses to achieve therapeutic effects.

Physiological factors, including age, body mass, organ function (especially liver and kidney function), and comorbid conditions, also play pivotal roles. These factors can alter drug absorption, distribution, metabolism, and excretion, necessitating dosage adjustments to achieve the desired drug concentration in the bloodstream.

Environmental and lifestyle factors, such as diet, smoking status, alcohol consumption, and adherence to medication regimens, further influence individual drug response. Certain foods and lifestyle habits can induce or inhibit the activity of drug-metabolizing enzymes, affecting drug levels and efficacy.

Understanding and anticipating individual response is a cornerstone of personalized medicine. It allows healthcare providers to tailor medication dosages more precisely, moving beyond one-size-fits-all approaches to consider the unique characteristics of each patient. This personalized strategy aims to maximize therapeutic benefits while minimizing risks, ensuring that medication management is as effective and safe as possible for every individual.

## Conclusion

These factors underscore the importance of personalized medicine, where dosages are tailored to the individual's specific characteristics and circumstances, ensuring both safety and efficacy in treatment.

# FOURTEEN
## Fundoplications

## Fundoplication

*Fundoplication* is a surgical procedure that aims to address *gastroesophageal reflux disease (GERD)*, a condition where stomach acid frequently flows back into the esophagus, causing irritation and symptoms such as heartburn. This procedure is also employed in the treatment of *hiatal hernias*, which can contribute to *GERD* symptoms. *Fundoplication* is often considered when lifestyle modifications and medications fail to adequately control *GERD* symptoms, offering a potential long-term solution for patients suffering from this condition.

## How does Fundoplication work?

Fundoplication involves wrapping the top part of the stomach (the fundus) around the *esophagus* and sewing it into place. This increases the pressure at the lower end of the *esophagus*, preventing acid reflux. The surgery can be performed using a *laparoscopic approach*, which involves making small incisions in the abdomen and using special instruments to complete the wrap, or through traditional open surgery with a larger incision.

The **Nissen fundoplication** is the most common type, where the stomach is wrapped 360 degrees around the *esophagus*. Partial wraps, like the **Toupet** (270 degrees) and **Dor** (180-200 degrees) fundoplications, are alternatives that might be used depending on the patient's specific situation.

# Benefits of Fundoplication

## Symptom Relief

The primary benefit of *fundoplication* is the significant reduction or complete elimination of *GERD* symptoms, including heartburn, regurgitation, and difficulty swallowing. By reinforcing the *lower esophageal sphincter (LES)*, fundoplication prevents the ascent of stomach acids, directly addressing the cause of discomfort. Patients often experience immediate and sustained relief from the chronic symptoms that have impacted their quality of life, enabling a return to normal activities without the constant worry of acid reflux episodes.

## Decreased Dependence on Medications

Many patients with Heartburn/*GERD* rely on daily medications, such as *proton pump inhibitors (PPIs)*, to manage their symptoms. While effective, these medications can have side effects and may lose efficacy over time. Fundoplication can reduce or eliminate the need for these medications, freeing patients from the costs and potential side effects associated with long-term pharmaceutical treatment.

## Prevention of Complications

*GERD* can lead to complications, including *esophagitis* (inflammation of the esophagus), *Barrett's esophagus* (a precancerous condition), and *esophageal strictures* (narrowing of the esophagus). Fundoplication reduces the risk of these complications by preventing acid reflux, thus offering a protective effect against the progression of GERD to more serious conditions.

## Improvement in Quality of Life

The discomfort and lifestyle limitations imposed by *GERD* can significantly affect a patient's quality of life. By effectively managing or eliminating symptoms, fundoplication allows individuals to enjoy meals without the fear of subsequent pain, sleep better without the discomfort of nighttime reflux, and engage in a wider range of activities. This improvement in quality of life is often cited by patients as a key benefit of the surgery.

## Durability of Treatment

Unlike medication, which must be taken daily to manage symptoms, fundoplication offers a long-term solution to *GERD*. When performed successfully, the benefits of the procedure can last for many years, providing patients with sustained relief and a significant reduction in the recurrence of symptoms.

## Minimal Invasiveness

With advancements in surgical techniques, fundoplication is often performed *laparoscopically*, involving only small incisions. This minimally invasive approach reduces recovery time, minimizes pain and scarring, and lowers the risk of complications associated with open surgery. Patients can typically return to their normal routines more quickly than with traditional surgery.

In conclusion, fundoplication presents a comprehensive solution for patients suffering from *GERD*, offering immediate and lasting symptom relief, a decrease in the need for medication, prevention of further esophageal damage, and a significant enhancement in overall quality of life. This procedure represents a turning point for many, providing them with the opportunity to lead a life free from the constraints of chronic acid reflux.

## Why does Fundoplication work?

The effectiveness of *fundoplication* lies in its ability to reconstruct the *LES's* barrier function. By wrapping the stomach around the *esophagus*, it effectively creates a new valve mechanism that can prevent the backflow of stomach acid. This mechanical enhancement to the *LES* augments its pressure, ensuring that it remains closed when not swallowing, thereby preventing acid reflux.

## Risks and Complications

While *fundoplication* is generally safe, like any surgery, it comes with potential risks and complications. These can include difficulty swallowing (*dysphagia*), gas-bloat syndrome, where patients have trouble belching or vomiting, and potential slippage of the stomach wrap over time. Other risks involve surgical complications such as infection, bleeding, or issues related to anesthesia. It's also possible for *GERD* symptoms to persist or recur after surgery, necessitating further medical intervention.

## The Surgical Process

Patients considering fundoplication undergo a comprehensive preoperative evaluation, including diagnostic tests like *endoscopy, esophageal manometry,* and pH monitoring. These assessments help confirm the diagnosis of *GERD*, evaluate the severity of the condition, and determine the esophagus's overall function to ensure the patient is a suitable candidate for surgery.

The procedure itself, especially when performed *laparoscopically,* typically involves a shorter hospital stay and recovery period compared to open surgery. Most patients can return to normal activities within a few weeks, although dietary restrictions are common immediately post-surgery to allow healing.

## Postoperative Care and Recovery

After *fundoplication*, patients may need to follow a phased diet beginning with liquids and gradually introducing soft then solid foods. This careful approach helps avoid putting undue pressure on the newly formed valve. Regular follow-up appointments are crucial to monitor recovery and address any complications.

## Rewards and Considerations

For many patients, fundoplication offers significant relief from *GERD* symptoms, allowing them to enjoy a higher quality of life without the constant discomfort of acid reflux. The reduction in the need for ongoing medication use and the prevention of long-term complications associated with *GERD* are notable benefits.

However, the decision to undergo *fundoplication* should be made after careful consideration of the potential risks and benefits. Discussion with a healthcare provider is essential to ensure that this surgical option is the best course of action for the individual's specific condition and overall health.

## Long-term Outcomes

Long-term studies on fundoplication report that the majority of patients experience a significant reduction in *GERD* symptoms and are satisfied with their surgical outcomes. While the procedure does not guarantee that *GERD* symptoms will never return, it significantly reduces the likelihood and severity of symptoms for many years post-surgery.

In conclusion, fundoplication represents a significant advancement in the treatment of GERD, offering hope and relief to those for whom conventional treatments have failed. By addressing the mechanical cause of *GERD*, fundoplication can effectively reduce or eliminate symptoms, improve quality of life, and prevent the progression of GERD-related complications. As with any medical procedure, individuals considering fundoplication should engage in open and informed discussions with their healthcare providers to thoroughly understand the potential risks and rewards.

~~~~~~~~~~~~~~~~~~~~~~~~~~~~~~~~~~~~~~~~

# 3 Types of Fundoplication Surgeries

~~~~~~~~~~~~~~~~~~~~~~~~~~~~~~~~~~~~~~~~

## Nissen Fundoplication (full wrap):

*The Nissen Fundoplication* is the most common of the three wrap surgeries. The procedure involves wrapping the top part of the stomach (the *fundus*) around the lower end of the *esophagus* and securing it in place. This effectively increases the pressure at the *lower esophageal sphincter (LES)*, the valve that naturally prevents stomach contents from moving upwards. By enhancing the integrity and function of the *LES*, the *Nissen fundoplication* reduces or eliminates the occurrence of acid reflux.

## How It Works

*Nissen fundoplication* can be performed through open surgery or more commonly now, via *laparoscopy*, which is minimally invasive. Laparoscopic surgery involves making small incisions in the abdomen through which surgical tools and a camera are inserted. This method reduces recovery time, scarring, and the risk of complications compared to open surgery.

## Pros of Nissen Fundoplication

- 1. **Effective in Reducing *GERD* Symptoms:** For many patients, Nissen fundoplication significantly reduces or completely eliminates symptoms of *GERD*, improving quality of life.
- 2. **Long-term Solution:** Unlike medication that requires ongoing use, Nissen fundoplication offers a long-term solution to GERD, with many patients experiencing relief for years after the surgery.
- 3. **Minimally Invasive Option:** When performed *laparoscopically*, the procedure is minimally invasive, leading to shorter hospital stays, quicker recovery times, and less postoperative pain.

- 4. **Reduces Dependence on Medications:** Patients often can reduce or eliminate the use of acid-suppressing medications, avoiding their costs and potential side effects.

## Cons of Nissen Fundoplication

- 1. **Surgical Risks:** As with any surgery, there are risks of complications, such as infection, bleeding, or damage to surrounding organs. Though rare, these risks should be considered.
- 2. **Difficulty Swallowing (*Dysphagia*):** Some patients may experience difficulty swallowing due to the tightness of the wrap around the *esophagus*. This is usually temporary but can be persistent in some cases.
- 3. **Gas-bloat Syndrome:** The procedure can make it difficult for some patients to belch or vomit, leading to discomfort from trapped gas in the stomach or bloating.
- 4. **Potential for Reoperation:** In some instances, the wrap may become loose or move, necessitating further surgery. Also, if the initial procedure was not effective, additional interventions might be required.

## Conclusion

*Nissen fundoplication* is a proven surgical approach to treating *GERD* and *hiatal hernias*, offering significant benefits for patients who have not found relief through medication or other treatments. While it has its advantages, including effectiveness and the potential for a long-term solution, it also carries risks and possible side effects. Patients considering this surgery should discuss the potential outcomes, risks, and benefits with their healthcare provider to make an informed decision that aligns with their health needs and lifestyle.

## Toupet Fundoplication (partial wrap):

*Toupet Fundoplication*, unlike the *Nissen fundoplication*, which wraps the stomach 360 degrees around the esophagus, the Toupet technique involves a 270-degree posterior wrap. This method is often recommended for patients with **esophageal motility disorders** or those who might not tolerate a full Nissen wrap due to its tighter constriction.

## How It Works

The Toupet fundoplication is primarily performed *laparoscopically*, involving small incisions in the abdomen through which surgical instruments and a camera are inserted. The surgeon partially wraps the fundus of the stomach around the back of the *esophagus* and sutures it in place. This action supports the *lower esophageal sphincter (LES)*, helping it prevent the reflux of gastric contents into the *esophagus*.

# Pros of Toupet Fundoplication

- 1. **Reduced Risk of *Dysphagia***: Compared to the *Nissen fundoplication*, patients undergoing Toupet fundoplication report fewer issues with *dysphagia* (difficulty swallowing) post-surgery due to the partial wrap.
- 2. **Effective *GERD* Management**: Toupet fundoplication is effective in reducing or eliminating GERD symptoms, offering significant relief to patients.
- 3. **Minimally Invasive**: Like the Nissen procedure, the Toupet is often performed *laparoscopically*, resulting in shorter recovery times, less postoperative pain, and minimal scarring.
- 4. **Suitable for Patients with Esophageal Motility Disorders**: This technique is preferred for patients who have diminished *esophageal motility*, as it imposes less pressure on the esophagus than a full wrap.

# Cons of Toupet Fundoplication

- 1. **Potential for Recurrence of Reflux**: Some studies suggest that the partial wrap might have a slightly higher rate of reflux recurrence compared to the full *Nissen wrap*.
- 2. **Surgical Risks**: As with any surgical procedure, there are inherent risks, including infection,

bleeding, and the possibility of damage to surrounding organs.

- 3. **Gas-bloat Syndrome:** Patients may still experience symptoms related to difficulty in belching or vomiting, leading to bloating and discomfort, although this is generally less severe than with the Nissen procedure.

## Conclusion

*The Toupet fundoplication* offers a valuable surgical option for managing *GERD*, particularly for patients with *esophageal motility* issues or those at risk of postoperative *dysphagia*. While it shares many of the advantages of the *Nissen fundoplication*, including effectiveness in reducing GERD symptoms and a minimally invasive approach, it also presents a unique set of considerations regarding the potential for reflux recurrence and surgical risks. Patients should engage in thorough discussions with their healthcare providers to determine the most appropriate treatment strategy based on their specific medical condition and lifestyle needs.

## Dor Fundoplication (partial anterior wrap):

*Dor Fundoplication*, also known as the anterior 180-degree wrap, is a surgical procedure employed to treat *gastroesophageal reflux disease (GERD)* and *hiatal hernias*. Unlike the *Nissen (360–degree wrap)* and *Toupet (270–degree wrap)* fundoplications, the *Dor* technique involves wrapping the front portion of the stomach around the lower part of the e*sophagus* and securing it, forming a partial wrap that reinforces the *lower esophageal sphincter (LES)* from the front. This method is often chosen for patients undergoing surgery for a *hiatal hernia* or those with compromised *esophageal motility* where a full wrap might exacerbate symptoms such as *dysphagia*.

# How It Works

Performed typically through *laparoscopic* surgery to minimize invasiveness, the *Dor fundoplication* involves folding the stomach's *fundus* around the anterior (front) side of the *esophagus* and suturing it in place. This configuration enhances the pressure at the *LES*, preventing the backflow of stomach acids into the esophagus, thereby reducing *GERD* symptoms.

## Pros of Dor Fundoplication

- 1. **Reduced Risk of *Dysphagia*:** The partial wrap is less likely to cause postoperative *dysphagia* compared to the *full Nissen wrap*, making it a suitable option for patients with swallowing difficulties.
- 2. **Effective Symptom Relief:** Dor fundoplication can significantly alleviate *GERD* symptoms, improving patients' quality of life.
- 3. **Minimally Invasive Approach:** When performed *laparoscopically*, the procedure entails a quicker

recovery, reduced pain, and fewer complications than open surgery.

## Cons of Dor Fundoplication

- 1. **Potential for Recurrence:** There might be a higher chance of *GERD* symptoms recurring compared to the Nissen fundoplication due to the less extensive wrap.
- 2. **Surgical Risks:** Despite being minimally invasive, risks such as infection, bleeding, and injury to surrounding organs exist.
- 3. **Gas-bloat Syndrome:** Patients may experience bloating and discomfort due to the inability to belch or vomit, similar to other *fundoplication* procedures, albeit potentially to a lesser extent.

## <u>Final thoughts on Fundoplication Surgery</u>

Deciding whether to undergo fundoplication surgery for the treatment of *gastroesophageal reflux disease (GERD)* or a *hiatal hernia* involves careful consideration of the benefits and risks associated with the procedure. Fundoplication, which can be performed using various techniques such as *Nissen, Toupet, or Dor*, aims to reinforce the lower esophageal sphincter (*LES*) to prevent the backflow of stomach acids into the *esophagus*, thereby alleviating symptoms of GERD and preventing further esophageal damage.

## Who Should Consider Fundoplication Surgery?

Individuals who should consider fundoplication surgery typically include those with severe *GERD* symptoms that have not responded to lifestyle changes or medication, those experiencing complications from GERD such as *esophagitis* or *Barrett's esophagus*, and those with a *hiatal hernia* causing significant symptoms or complications. It's also considered for patients who wish to avoid long-term medication use due to side effects or costs.

## Benefits vs. Risks

The benefits of fundoplication include long-term relief from *GERD* symptoms, reduction or elimination of the need for GERD medications, and prevention of GERD-related complications. However, potential risks include surgical complications, difficulty swallowing (*dysphagia*), gas-bloat syndrome, and the possibility of needing additional surgeries if the wrap loosens or becomes ineffective over time.

## Conclusion

The decision to undergo fundoplication should be made after thorough discussions with a healthcare provider, considering the severity of symptoms, response to other treatments, and individual patient preferences and health conditions. While fundoplication offers a potentially effective long-term solution for *GERD*, it is not suitable for everyone. Evaluating the balance between the procedure's benefits and risks is crucial in making an informed decision that aligns with one's health goals and quality of life expectations.

# LINX Device

The *LINX Device* is a revolutionary approach to treating *gastroesophageal reflux disease (GERD)*, which causes symptoms like heartburn, regurgitation, and potential damage to the esophagus lining. Unlike traditional surgical treatments like *Nissen or Toupet fundoplication*, the LINX system involves the placement of a small, flexible band of magnetic titanium beads around the *lower esophageal sphincter (LES)*. This innovative procedure aims to strengthen the LES, preventing acid reflux while allowing normal swallowing and digestion.

## How It Works

The LINX device is implanted *laparoscopically*, meaning through minimally invasive surgery, under *general anesthesia*. The band is positioned around the outside of the *esophagus* just above the stomach, at the site of the *LES*. The magnetic beads are strong enough to keep the LES closed to refluxing acid but will temporarily separate to allow food and liquid to pass into the stomach. The device is designed to support the LES's natural barrier function against reflux while not disrupting normal esophageal and gastric functions such as swallowing, belching, and vomiting.

## Pros of the LINX Device

- 1. **Effectiveness:** The LINX device has been shown to significantly reduce or eliminate *GERD* symptoms in a majority of patients, improving their quality of life.
- 2. **Minimally Invasive Procedure:** The surgery is performed *laparoscopically*, which typically results in shorter hospital stays, faster recovery times, and less postoperative pain compared to traditional open surgeries.
- 3. **Preservation of Stomach Anatomy:** Unlike *fundoplication*, which involves wrapping the stomach around the *esophagus*, the LINX procedure does not alter the stomach anatomy, which could lead to fewer long-term complications.
- 4. **Reversible:** If necessary, the device can be surgically removed, and the procedure is reversible, which is not always the case with traditional fundoplication surgeries.

# Cons of the LINX Device

- 1. **Surgical Risks:** As with any surgical procedure, there are inherent risks such as infection, bleeding, adverse reactions to anesthesia, and potential injury to surrounding tissues.
- 2. **Dysphagia:** Some patients may experience difficulty swallowing (*dysphagia*) after the procedure, although this is usually temporary and often resolves within a few weeks to months post-surgery.
- 3. **Foreign Body Sensation:** Patients may feel a sensation of having a foreign body in their throat, especially in the initial period after the implantation.
- 4. **Magnetic Interference:** The magnetic beads could potentially interact with magnetic fields, including those from MRI machines. Patients with a *LINX device* are advised to avoid certain types of MRI scans or may require a specific kind of MRI.
- 5. **Long-term Efficacy and Complications:** While the LINX device has shown promising results, it is a relatively new treatment option compared to traditional surgeries. Long-term data on efficacy and potential complications are still being gathered.

# Conclusion

The LINX device offers a novel and effective treatment option for patients with *GERD*, particularly for those who have not achieved sufficient relief from medication or are seeking an alternative to more invasive surgical procedures like fundoplication. Its minimally invasive nature, combined with the preservation of stomach anatomy and the possibility of reversal, makes it an attractive option for many.

However, potential candidates for the LINX procedure must carefully weigh the benefits against the risks, including the possibility of *dysphagia*, the need to avoid certain MRIs, and the long-term performance of the device. As with any medical treatment, discussions with a healthcare provider specializing in *GERD* management are crucial to determine the most appropriate option based on individual symptoms, lifestyle, and health goals

# Heartburn Healing Final Thoughts

As we come to the end of this journey together, I want to express my sincere hope that the information within these pages has become an inspiring light, guiding you towards relief from the discomfort of heartburn.

Throughout our exploration, we've looked at  the profound importance of stomach acid for our overall well-being. Rather than seeking to eliminate it entirely, we've grasped the idea of harmonizing with it through mindful, healthful choices in diet and lifestyle.

I trust that you've discovered a wealth of remedies, both traditional and innovative, that resonate with your unique needs. From the comforting embrace of herbal remedies to the empowering support of dietary supplements, the possibilities are boundless. And who knows? Maybe you've come across a handful of unique solutions that make perfect sense to you.

For those who still require medications, I trust that you now have a more comprehensive grasp of the extensive variety of options that exist, empowering you to make informed decisions that align with your personal health journey.

As you venture forth into the future, equipped with comprehensive wisdom and anchored in practicality, I encourage you to embrace the impact of these methodologies. Let them serve as the foundation upon which you build a life of greater vitality and joy.

Walk forward with confidence, knowing that each choice you make brings you one step closer to a brighter, healthier future. You deserve nothing less than to thrive, and I believe wholeheartedly that you have the resilience and determination to do just that.

Here's to living healthier and happier, one mindful decision at a time.

With boundless hope and unwavering support,

Lillian Heart ♡

# Quick Reference Guide

## Foods That Can Cause Heartburn

- ☐ Spicy foods (e.g., hot peppers, chili)
- ☐ Citrus fruits (e.g., oranges, grapefruits, lemons)
- ☐ Tomatoes and tomato-based products (e.g., tomato sauce, ketchup)
- ☐ Chocolate
- ☐ Fatty or fried foods
- ☐ Onions
- ☐ Garlic
- ☐ Peppermint and mint-flavored foods
- ☐ Vinegar and vinegar-based dressings
- ☐ High-fat dairy products (e.g., cheese, cream)
- ☐ Processed meats (e.g., bacon, sausage, deli meats)
- ☐ Spicy condiments (e.g., hot sauce, mustard)
- ☐ Fried foods (e.g., french fries, fried chicken)
- ☐ Acidic fruits (e.g., pineapple, berries)
- ☐ High-sugar foods (e.g., candies, sweets)
- ☐ High-fat desserts (e.g., ice cream, pastries)

☐ Tomato-based condiments (e.g., salsa, marinara sauce)

☐ Peppers (e.g., bell peppers, chili peppers)

☐ Mustard and mustard-based condiments

☐ Processed snacks (e.g., chips, crackers)

☐ Fried or greasy snacks (e.g., potato chips, cheese puffs)

☐ Pizza

☐ Burgers

☐ Tacos

☐ Burritos

☐ Nachos

☐ Enchiladas

☐ Chili con carne

☐ Spaghetti and meatballs

☐ Lasagna

☐ Cheeseburgers

☐ Fried chicken sandwiches

☐ Hot dogs

☐ Fried seafood (e.g., shrimp, calamari)

☐ Cheese-filled dishes (e.g., stuffed crust pizza, cheese-filled pasta)

- ☐ Cheesy dips and sauces (e.g., queso dip, cheese fondue)
- ☐ Cream-based soups (e.g., clam chowder, cream of mushroom soup)
- ☐ Creamy pasta dishes (e.g., fettuccine Alfredo, macaroni and cheese)
- ☐ Butter-rich dishes (e.g., buttery croissants, buttery mashed potatoes)
- ☐ Heavy gravies and sauces (e.g., sausage gravy, hollandaise sauce)
- ☐ Creamy desserts (e.g., cheesecake, chocolate mousse)
- ☐ Ice cream sundaes
- ☐ Puddings and custards
- ☐ Rich pastries (e.g., croissants, Danish pastries)
- ☐ Donuts
- ☐ Cream-filled cakes (e.g., Boston cream pie, éclairs)
- ☐ Buttery cookies (e.g., shortbread cookies, butter cookies)
- ☐ Deep-fried desserts (e.g., funnel cakes, churros)
- ☐ Creamy dips (e.g., spinach artichoke dip, buffalo chicken dip)

☐ Rich chocolate desserts (e.g., chocolate lava cake, chocolate truffles)

# Beverages That Can Cause Heartburn

☐ Coffee (both regular and decaffeinated)

☐ Tea (black, green, and some herbal teas)

☐ Carbonated drinks (e.g., soda, sparkling water)

☐ Alcohol (especially red wine)

☐ White wine

☐ Beer

☐ Spirits (e.g., whiskey, vodka, rum)

☐ Champagne

☐ Cocktails with citrus juices or spicy ingredients

☐ Citrus juices (e.g., orange juice, lemonade)

☐ Tomato juice

☐ Cranberry juice

☐ Grapefruit juice

☐ Pineapple juice

☐ Lemon water or lemonade

☐ Lime water or limeade

☐ Spicy cocktails (e.g., Bloody Mary)

- ☐ Hot chocolate
- ☐ Chocolate milk
- ☐ Energy drinks
- ☐ Sports drinks
- ☐ Carbonated energy drinks
- ☐ Carbonated mixed drinks (e.g., rum and cola)
- ☐ Coffee-based drinks (e.g., lattes, mochas)
- ☐ Tea-based drinks (e.g., sweet tea, chai lattes)
- ☐ Milkshakes
- ☐ Smoothies with citrus fruits or high acidity
- ☐ Milk (for some individuals)
- ☐ Soy milk (for some individuals)
- ☐ Almond milk (for some individuals)
- ☐ Coconut milk (for some individuals)
- ☐ Oat milk (for some individuals)
- ☐ Rice milk (for some individuals)
- ☐ Hemp milk (for some individuals)
- ☐ Flavored milk alternatives (e.g., chocolate almond milk)
- ☐ Hot cider
- ☐ Mulled wine
- ☐ Eggnog

- ☐ Tonic water

- ☐ Carbonated lemonades or fruit-flavored sodas

- ☐ Carbonated ginger ale or ginger beer

- ☐ Flavored water with added citrus or spices

- ☐ Spicy tomato-based drinks

- ☐ Herbal teas with citrus or spicy ingredients

- ☐ Some fruit-flavored herbal teas

- ☐ Peppermint tea

- ☐ Spearmint tea

- ☐ Chai tea

- ☐ Spicy cinnamon teas (e.g., ginger, turmeric, licorice, chamomile, fennel and hibiscus)

# Overview of Medication Approaches

As extensively discussed earlier, each remedy for heartburn has its unique mechanism of action, benefits, and potential drawbacks. Here's a summarized comparison and contrast based on their effectiveness, usage, and side effects:

## Antacids

- *Mechanism*: Neutralize stomach acid on contact.
- *Use*: Immediate, short-term relief of mild heartburn and indigestion.
- **Pros**: Quick relief, over-the-counter availability, variety of forms.
- **Cons**: Short duration of effect, potential for rebound acidity, may interfere with the absorption of other medications.

## H2 Blockers

- *Mechanism*: Reduce acid production by blocking *histamine* receptors in stomach lining.
- *Use*: Longer-lasting relief than antacids, used for mild to moderate *GERD*.
- **Pros**: Longer duration of action than antacids, available OTC and in prescription strength.

- **Cons**: Slower onset of relief compared to antacids, potential for tolerance with long-term use.

# Proton Pump Inhibitors (PPIs)

- *Mechanism*: Block the enzyme necessary for acid secretion, providing more sustained acid suppression.
- *Use*: Treatment of moderate to severe *GERD*, *peptic ulcers*, and for long-term GERD management.
- **Pros**: Provides long-lasting relief, effective for healing *erosive esophagitis*.
- **Cons**: Risk of long-term side effects (e.g., nutrient deficiencies, increased risk of infections), delayed onset of relief.

# Prokinetics

- *Mechanism*: Enhance gastric emptying and *esophageal motility*.
- *Use*: Used when *GERD* is associated with delayed gastric emptying.
- **Pros**: Addresses underlying motility issues, complements acid suppression therapies.
- **Cons**: Limited availability due to side effects, may not directly relieve heartburn.

# Alginates

- *Mechanism*: Form a viscous barrier floating on the stomach contents, preventing reflux.
- *Use*: Symptomatic relief of *GERD*, particularly ***postprandial heartburn***.
- **Pros**: Quick relief, acts physically rather than altering acid chemistry.
- **Cons**: May need frequent dosing, effectiveness varies with stomach contents.

# Coating Agents

- *Mechanism*: Coat the stomach lining or ulcer sites, protecting them from acid.
- *Use*: Protection of ulcers, management of mild esophageal irritation.
- **Pros**: Provides a protective barrier, beneficial for patients with ulcers.
- **Cons**: Does not reduce acid production, limited to symptom management.

# Comparison:

Antacids and alginates offer quick, symptomatic relief but don't address the root cause of heartburn. H2 blockers and PPIs reduce acid production, with PPIs offering the most potent and longest-lasting relief but with a higher risk of long-term side effects. Prokinetics offer a different approach by enhancing motility, useful in specific cases but with limited application due to potential side effects. Coating agents, like alginates, provide a protective barrier, beneficial for symptom management and protection of the gastrointestinal lining but without affecting acid production.

# Conclusion:

Choosing the right heartburn remedy depends on the severity and frequency of symptoms, individual health conditions, and potential side effects.

For occasional, mild heartburn, antacids or alginates may suffice. For chronic or severe cases, PPIs are often the most effective option, though long-term use requires careful consideration and monitoring. H2 blockers represent a middle ground, offering significant relief with fewer risks than PPIs. Prokinetics and coating agents have niche roles, addressing specific aspects of digestive health. Always consult with a healthcare professional to determine the most appropriate treatment for your needs.

# Glossary of Terms

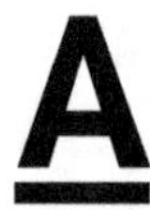

**Acetylcholine** - A neurotransmitter that facilitates communication between nerves and muscles and is involved in memory and learning.

**Acid Indigestion** - Discomfort in the stomach caused by the irritation of the digestive tract with too much acid, leading to symptoms like heartburn.

**Acid Reflux** - Acid reflux is a condition where stomach acid flows back into the esophagus, causing irritation and heartburn.

**Acidosis** - A condition characterized by excessive acidity in the body's fluids, leading to a lower than normal blood pH level.

**Aciphex** - A Proton Pump Inhibitor (PPI) medication used to treat acid reflux, gastroesophageal reflux disease (GERD), and ulcers by reducing stomach acid production. May Contain: Rabeprazole.

**Acupressure wristbands** - Wearable devices designed to apply pressure to specific points on the wrist, believed to relieve nausea and vomiting.

**Acupuncture** - A traditional Chinese medical practice that involves inserting thin needles into specific points on the body to relieve pain and treat various health conditions.

**Acute Interstitial Nephritis** - A kidney disorder involving inflammation of the kidney's interstitial tissue, leading to reduced kidney function and often caused by allergic reactions to medications.

**Adenocarcinoma** - A type of cancer that forms in mucus-secreting glands throughout the body, commonly affecting organs like the lungs, breasts, colon, and prostate.

**Adipose Tissue** - A type of body fat that stores energy, insulates the body, and cushions and protects organs.

**Alginates** - Natural polysaccharides extracted from seaweed, used in medical products for wound dressings and as thickening agents in food.

**Alka-Seltzer Heartburn Relief** - An Antacid, over-the-counter effervescent tablet designed to neutralize stomach acid, providing quick relief from heartburn and indigestion. May Contain: Sodium Bicarbonate and Calcium Carbonate.

**Aloe Vera Juice** - A liquid made from the pulp of the aloe vera plant, often used for its digestive, skin-healing, and anti-inflammatory properties.

**Aloe Vera Plant** - The Aloe Vera plant is a succulent known for its medicinal properties, including soothing skin irritations, burns, and supporting digestive health.

**Althaea Officinalis Plant** - (or marshmallow plant), a perennial herb known for its mucilaginous properties used in treating sore throats, coughs, and digestive issues.

**Aluminum Hydroxide** - An Antacid medication, used to neutralize stomach acid and alleviate symptoms of heartburn, indigestion, and upset stomach. It works by reducing acidity in the stomach (page 202, 207).

**Amino Acids** - Organic compounds that serve as the building blocks for proteins, crucial for various bodily functions including tissue repair, nutrient absorption, and muscle growth.

**Anecdotal** - Refers to information based on personal accounts or observations rather than scientific analysis or empirical evidence.

**Anemia** - A condition characterized by a deficiency of red blood cells or hemoglobin in the blood, leading to fatigue and weakness.

**Anethole** - A natural organic compound with a sweet, licorice-like flavor, primarily found in anise, fennel, and other plants, used as a flavoring agent.

**Antacid** - A medication that neutralizes stomach acid to relieve heartburn, acid indigestion, and stomach upset. May contain Magnesium Hydroxide, Aluminum Hydroxide, Calcium Carbonate, and Sodium Bicarbonate.

**Antiemetic Effect** - Refers to the ability of a substance to prevent or reduce nausea and vomiting.

**Anticoagulants** - Medications that prevent blood clot formation, reducing the risk of stroke, heart attack, and deep vein thrombosis.

**Antifungals** - Medications used to treat fungal infections by inhibiting the growth of fungi or killing them outright.

**Antihistamines** - Medications that block the action of histamine, reducing allergy symptoms such as itching, sneezing, and runny nose.

**Antimicrobial Properties** - Refer to the ability of a substance to inhibit the growth or kill microorganisms such as bacteria, viruses, and fungi.

**Antioxidant Properties** - Refer to the ability of a substance to neutralize harmful molecules called free radicals, thereby reducing oxidative stress and protecting cells from damage.

**Antispasmodic Properties** - Refer to the ability of a substance to relax and reduce muscle spasms or contractions.

**Apple Cider Vinegar (ACV)** - A fermented liquid made from crushed apples, often used in folk medicine for its potential health benefits and culinary purposes.

**Aromatherapy** - A holistic healing practice that uses natural plant extracts, known as essential oils, to promote physical, emotional, and mental well-being through inhalation or topical application.

**Arrhythmias** - Irregular heart rhythms that can manifest as too fast, too slow, or irregular heartbeats, potentially leading to palpitations, dizziness, or fainting.

**Asanas** - Physical postures or poses practiced in yoga to promote flexibility, strength, and relaxation.

**Aspiration Pneumonia** - A lung infection that occurs when foreign material, such as food, saliva, or vomit, is inhaled into the lungs, leading to inflammation and infection.

**Asthma Exacerbations** - Refer to worsening symptoms of asthma, such as coughing, wheezing, and shortness of breath, often triggered by factors like allergies, respiratory infections, or exposure to irritants.

**Axid AR** - An H2 Blocker over-the-counter medication used to treat heartburn and acid reflux by reducing stomach acid production. May Contain: Nizatidine.

# B

**Bacteria** - Single-celled microorganisms found in various environments, some of which can cause infections and diseases in humans.

**Barium Swallow Studies** - Diagnostic tests where a patient swallows a contrast material containing barium, allowing X-rays to visualize the esophagus, stomach, and upper gastrointestinal tract for abnormalities.

**Barrett's Esophagus** - A condition where the lining of the esophagus changes, increasing the risk of developing esophageal cancer.

**BHA** - (or Butylated hydroxyanisole), a synthetic antioxidant commonly used as a food preservative to prevent rancidity and extend shelf life.

**BHT** - (or Butylated hydroxytoluene), a synthetic antioxidant often used as a food preservative to prevent oxidation and extend shelf life.

**Bicarbonate** - A chemical compound that acts as a buffer in the body, helping to maintain the pH balance of bodily fluids and regulate acid-base levels.

**Bile** - A fluid produced by the liver and stored in the gallbladder, which aids in digestion by emulsifying fats and facilitating their absorption in the small intestine.

**Bioactive** - Refers to substances or compounds that have a specific biological effect on living organisms, often exerting beneficial effects on health or physiological functions.

**Bioequivalence** - Refers to the similarity in the rate and extent of absorption of a drug product compared to a reference product, indicating comparable effectiveness and safety profiles.

**Biopsies** - Medical procedures where small tissue samples are taken from the body for examination under a microscope to diagnose or monitor diseases such as cancer.

**Biopsy** - A medical procedure involving the removal of a small tissue sample from the body for examination under a microscope to diagnose or evaluate a disease.

**Bismuth Subsalicylate** - A Coating Agent medication, used to treat nausea, heartburn, indigestion, upset stomach, and diarrhea. It coats the stomach lining and has antimicrobial properties (page 293).

**Bisphosphonates** - Medications used to treat osteoporosis and other bone disorders by inhibiting bone breakdown and increasing bone density.

**Bolus** - A single, concentrated dose of medication or substance administered rapidly, often intravenously, to achieve a desired therapeutic effect.

**Bronchial Hygiene Techniques** - Refer to various methods, such as chest physiotherapy and airway clearance devices, used to remove mucus and secretions from the airways to improve breathing and prevent infections in patients with respiratory conditions.

**Bronchoconstriction** - Narrowing of the airways in the lungs due to muscle contraction, leading to difficulty breathing and respiratory symptoms such as wheezing and chest tightness.

# C

**Calcium Carbonate** - An antacid medication and dietary supplement used to treat conditions like heartburn and indigestion by neutralizing stomach acid and providing calcium supplementation (page 196, 286).

**Calcium Ions** - Positively charged particles of calcium that play crucial roles in various physiological processes, including muscle contraction, nerve signaling, and bone formation.

**Capsaicin** - A natural compound found in chili peppers that produces a burning sensation when in contact with skin or mucous membranes, commonly used for pain relief and as a culinary spice.

**Carminative** - Substances that relieve gas and bloating by promoting the expulsion of gas from the digestive tract, often used to alleviate gastrointestinal discomfort.

**CCK** - (or Cholecystokinin), A hormone released by the small intestine in response to the presence of fats, proteins, and acids in the digestive tract, stimulating the release of digestive enzymes and bile from the pancreas and gallbladder, respectively.

**Chamomile Tea** - A herbal infusion made from dried chamomile flowers, known for its calming and soothing properties, often consumed to promote relaxation and alleviate stress.

**Chelated Compound** - A chemical complex formed when a metal ion is bound to a chelating agent, making it easier for the body to absorb and use effectively.

**Chemoreceptor Trigger Zone** - An area in the brain that detects toxic substances and triggers vomiting to expel them from the body.

**Chemotherapy** - A systemic treatment for cancer that involves the use of powerful drugs to kill cancer cells or prevent their proliferation. It works by targeting rapidly dividing cells, which includes both cancerous and healthy cells, leading to side effects such as nausea, hair loss, and weakened immune system.

**Chiropractic Care** - A healthcare approach that focuses on diagnosing and treating musculoskeletal disorders, primarily through manual adjustments and manipulations of the spine and other joints.

**Cholecystokinin** - (or CCK), A hormone released by the small intestine in response to the presence of fats, proteins, and acids in the digestive tract, stimulating the release of digestive enzymes and bile from the pancreas and gallbladder, respectively.

**Chronic Constipation** - A long-term condition characterized by infrequent bowel movements, difficulty passing stools, and/or incomplete evacuation, often causing discomfort and bloating.

**Chronic Cough** - A persistent cough lasting for more than eight weeks, often indicative of an underlying medical condition such as asthma, postnasal drip, or gastroesophageal reflux disease.

**Chronic Gastritis** - Long-term inflammation of the stomach lining, often leading to digestive symptoms such as abdominal pain, nausea, and vomiting.

**Chronic Idiopathic Constipation** - (or CIC), refers to long-term constipation with no identifiable cause, characterized by infrequent or difficult bowel movements and abdominal discomfort.

**Chronic Kidney Disease** - Long-term damage to the kidneys, leading to reduced kidney function and potential complications such as fluid retention and electrolyte imbalances.

**Chyme** - Semi-liquid mixture of partially digested food, gastric juices, and stomach acid that passes from the stomach to the small intestine during digestion.

**CIC** - (or Chronic idiopathic constipation), refers to long-term constipation with no identifiable cause, characterized by infrequent or difficult bowel movements and abdominal discomfort.

**Cimetidine** - An H2 Blocker medication that reduces stomach acid production, often prescribed for conditions like ulcers and GERD. It belongs to H2 receptor antagonists, alleviating symptoms such as heartburn and acid indigestion (page 218).

**Clostridium Difficile Infection** - A bacterial infection that causes diarrhea and inflammation of the colon, often occurring after antibiotic use disrupts the normal balance of gut bacteria.

**Coating Agents** - Medications that create a protective barrier on the lining of the gastrointestinal tract, helping to alleviate symptoms such as heartburn and ulcers by shielding the mucosa from irritation and acidity.

**Colitis** - Inflammation of the colon, leading to symptoms such as abdominal pain, diarrhea, and rectal bleeding, often caused by conditions like inflammatory bowel disease or infection.

**Colonic Motility** - Refers to the movement and contraction of muscles in the colon, facilitating the passage of stool through the digestive tract.

**Columnar Epithelium** - A type of tissue that lines the inside of organs, featuring tall cells arranged like columns, commonly found in the digestive system.

**Corticosteroids** - Medications that mimic the effects of hormones produced by the adrenal glands, often used to reduce inflammation and suppress the immune system in various medical conditions.

**Creatinine Clearance** - A measure of kidney function, calculated by comparing the amount of creatinine excreted in urine over a specific time period to the concentration of creatinine in the blood.

**CT Scans** - (or computed tomography scans), are medical imaging tests that use X-rays and computer processing to create detailed cross-sectional images of the body, aiding in diagnosis and treatment planning.

**CYP450 Enzyme Family** - A group of enzymes involved in the metabolism of various substances, including drugs, toxins, and hormones, within the body's cells.

**Cytochrome P450 Enzyme System** - A group of enzymes responsible for metabolizing drugs and other foreign compounds in the body, affecting their effectiveness and potential interactions.

**Cytokines** - Small proteins secreted by cells that regulate immune responses and inflammation, playing a crucial role in coordinating the body's defense against infections and diseases.

# D

**Deglycyrrhizinated Licorice** - (or DGL), A form of licorice root extract with the compound glycyrrhizin removed, often used to alleviate symptoms of heartburn, acid reflux, and stomach ulcers.

**Delayed Stomach Emptying** - Also known as gastroparesis, is a condition where the stomach takes longer than normal to empty its contents into the small intestine, leading to symptoms such as nausea, vomiting, and bloating.

**Denaturation** - A process in which the structure of a protein is altered, typically due to factors such as heat, pH changes, or chemical exposure, leading to loss of function.

**Dexilant** - A Proton Pump Inhibitor medication, used to treat gastroesophageal reflux disease (GERD) and related conditions by reducing stomach acid production. May Contain: Dexlansoprazole.

**Dexlansoprazole** - A proton pump inhibitor medication used to treat conditions like gastroesophageal reflux disease (GERD) and stomach ulcers by decreasing stomach acid production, relieving symptoms such as heartburn and acid reflux (page 249).

**DGL** - (or Deglycyrrhizinated licorice), a form of licorice root extract with the compound glycyrrhizin removed, often used to alleviate symptoms of heartburn, acid reflux, and stomach ulcers.

**Diaphragmatic Breathing** - A breathing technique that involves deep inhalation and expansion of the diaphragm, promoting relaxation and reducing stress by engaging the body's natural relaxation response.

**Digestive Enzymes** - Proteins produced by the body to break down food into smaller, absorbable nutrients, aiding in digestion and nutrient absorption in the gastrointestinal tract.

**Dipeptide** - A chemical compound consisting of two amino acids linked together by a peptide bond, forming the simplest unit of a peptide. These molecules play crucial roles in protein synthesis, digestion, and various physiological processes within living organisms.

**Diuretic** - A diuretic is a medication or substance that increases urine production, leading to increased excretion of water and electrolytes from the body.

**Domperidone** - A Pprokinetic medication used to treat gastrointestinal disorders by promoting gastric emptying and reducing nausea and vomiting (page 261).

**Dopamine Antagonist** - A medication that blocks the action of dopamine, often used to treat conditions such as psychosis, nausea, and certain neurological disorders.

**Dopamine Receptor Antagonist** - A medication that blocks dopamine receptors, commonly used to treat conditions like schizophrenia, nausea, and certain neurological disorders.

**Dopamine Receptors** - Proteins located on the surface of cells in the brain and other parts of the body that bind to the neurotransmitter dopamine, playing a key role in various physiological processes including mood regulation, movement, and reward pathways.

**Dor Fundoplication** - A surgical procedure to treat gastroesophageal reflux disease (GERD) by wrapping the upper part of the stomach around the lower esophagus to reinforce the barrier between the stomach and esophagus, reducing reflux.

**Duodenal Ulcers** - Sores or lesions that develop in the lining of the first part of the small intestine (duodenum), often caused by factors like H. pylori infection, NSAIDs, or excess stomach acid.

**Dysbiosis** - Refers to an imbalance or disruption in the normal microbial community (microbiota) of the gut, potentially leading to health problems or disease.

**Dyspepsia** - A medical term for discomfort or pain in the upper abdomen, often associated with symptoms like bloating, nausea, and early satiety, without a specific identifiable cause.

**Dysphagia** - Difficulty swallowing, often due to problems with the muscles or nerves involved in the swallowing process, which can occur as a result of surgery.

# E

**Electrolyte** - A substance that conducts electricity when dissolved in water and dissociates into ions, crucial for various physiological functions including nerve signaling, muscle contraction, and maintaining fluid balance.

**Electrolyte Imbalances** - Refer to disruptions in the levels of ions such as sodium, potassium, calcium, and chloride in the body, which can lead to health complications affecting vital functions like heart rhythm, nerve signaling, and muscle contraction.

**EMR** - (or Endoscopic Mucosal Resection) is a minimally invasive procedure to remove abnormal tissues or early-stage cancers from the digestive tract using an endoscope with specialized tools.

**Endorphins** - Neurotransmitters produced by the body that act as natural painkillers and contribute to feelings of pleasure and well-being.

**Endoscope** - A flexible or rigid tube with a light and camera used to visualize internal structures or organs in the body, often inserted through natural openings or small incisions for diagnostic or therapeutic purposes.

**Endoscopic Exams** - Involve the use of an endoscope to visually examine internal organs or structures for diagnostic or therapeutic purposes.

**Endoscopic Mucosal Resection** - (or EMR) is a minimally invasive procedure to remove abnormal tissues or early-stage cancers from the digestive tract using an endoscope with specialized tools.

**Endoscopy** - A medical procedure using an endoscope to visually examine the inside of the body for diagnostic or therapeutic purposes.

**Enteric Nervous System** - A complex network of nerves within the gastrointestinal tract responsible for regulating digestion, secretion, and motility, often referred to as the "second brain" of the body.

**Enzymatic Reactions** - Biochemical processes facilitated by enzymes, which catalyze the conversion of substrates into products, often essential for metabolic pathways and cellular functions.

**Enzymes** - Proteins that catalyze biochemical reactions, accelerating chemical processes in living organisms without being consumed themselves.

**Eosinophil** - A type of white blood cell involved in the immune response against parasites and allergic reactions, characterized by their large granules and nucleus shape.

**Eosinophilic Esophagitis** - A chronic inflammatory condition of the esophagus characterized by the presence of eosinophils, often triggered by allergic reactions to certain foods or environmental factors.

**Epithelialization** - Process of new epithelial cells migrating and proliferating to cover a wound or injury during the healing process, forming a protective barrier.

**Erosive Esophagitis** - inflammation and erosion of the lining of the esophagus, often caused by prolonged exposure to stomach acid due to gastroesophageal reflux disease (GERD).

**Esomeprazole** - A Proton Pump Inhibitor medication, commonly prescribed to alleviate symptoms of acid-related conditions like gastroesophageal reflux disease (GERD) and peptic ulcers by reducing stomach acid production (page 237).

**Esophageal Adenocarcinoma** - A type of cancer that originates in the cells lining the lower part of the esophagus, often associated with chronic gastroesophageal reflux disease (GERD) and Barrett's esophagus.

**Esophageal Cancer** - Malignancy that develops in the cells of the esophagus, often associated with risk factors like smoking, alcohol consumption, and gastroesophageal reflux disease (GERD).

**Esophageal Manometry** - A diagnostic test used to evaluate the function and motility of the esophagus by measuring the pressure exerted by the muscles in the esophageal wall during swallowing.

**Esophageal Motility Disorders** - Conditions characterized by abnormal contractions or movements of the muscles in the esophagus, leading to difficulties in swallowing and other symptoms.

**Esophageal Sphincter** - Muscular valve at the junction of the esophagus and stomach that controls the flow of food and prevents gastric reflux.

**Esophageal Stricture** - A narrowing of the esophagus often due to scar tissue formation, inflammation, or tumors, leading to difficulty swallowing and potentially causing food impaction.

**Esophageal Ulcers** - Sores or lesions that develop in the lining of the esophagus, typically caused by irritation from stomach acid reflux or certain medications.

**Esophagitis** - Inflammation of the lining of the esophagus, often caused by acid reflux, infections, or certain medications, leading to symptoms such as heartburn and difficulty swallowing.

**Esophagus** - The esophagus is a muscular tube in the digestive system that connects the throat to the stomach, facilitating the passage of food and liquids through peristaltic contractions.

**Estragole** - A natural compound found in certain plants and herbs, known for its aromatic properties, but it may pose health risks due to potential carcinogenic effects.

**Extrapyramidal Symptoms** - Involuntary movement disorders such as tremors, rigidity, and dystonia caused by dysfunction in the brain's extrapyramidal system, often as a side effect of certain medications.

# F

**Famotidine** - An H2 Blocker medication, commonly used to reduce stomach acid production and treat conditions such as ulcers, gastroesophageal reflux disease (GERD), and heartburn (page 215).

**FDA** - (or Food and Drug Administration), is a federal agency in the United States responsible for regulating and supervising food safety, pharmaceuticals, medical devices, cosmetics, and other products.

**Fenchone** - A natural compound found in various plants and herbs, known for its aromatic properties and sometimes used in traditional medicine for its potential therapeutic effects.

**Fennel** - A flowering plant with aromatic seeds and leaves, used in cooking and traditional medicine for its digestive and flavor-enhancing properties.

**Fermentation** - A metabolic process in which microorganisms like bacteria and yeast convert carbohydrates into alcohol, acids, or gasses, often used in food production and as a metabolic pathway in cells.

**Flavonoids** - A group of plant compounds with antioxidant properties, found in fruits, vegetables, and herbs, associated with various health benefits such as reducing inflammation and improving cardiovascular health.

**Flora** - Refers to the collective microorganisms, including bacteria, fungi, and other microbes, residing in or on a specific environment or organism, such as the gut flora in the digestive tract.

**Fundoplication** - A surgical procedure used to treat gastroesophageal reflux disease (GERD) by wrapping the upper part of the stomach around the lower esophagus to reinforce the barrier between the stomach and esophagus, reducing reflux.

**Fundus** - The upper portion or rounded part of an organ, typically used to refer to the top section of the stomach or the top of the uterus during pregnancy.

# G

**GALT** - (or Gut-Associated Lymphoid Tissue), a component of the immune system located in the gastrointestinal tract, comprising lymphoid cells and structures that defend against pathogens and maintain immune balance.

**Gasmotin** - A Prokinetic medication, primarily used to treat ulcers and gastroesophageal reflux disease (GERD) by reducing stomach acid production. May Contain: Mosapride Citrate.

**Gastric Acid** - A digestive fluid produced by the stomach that aids in the breakdown of food and helps to kill bacteria ingested with food.

**Gastric Secretion** - Refers to the production of digestive fluids, including gastric acid and enzymes, by the stomach's mucosal cells, essential for digestion and nutrient absorption.

**Gastric Ulcers** - Sores or lesions that develop in the lining of the stomach, often caused by factors like H. pylori infection, NSAIDs, or excess stomach acid.

**Gastrin** - A hormone produced by the stomach that stimulates the secretion of gastric acid, aiding in the digestion of food.

**Gastroenterologist** - A medical doctor who specializes in diagnosing and treating disorders of the digestive system, including the esophagus, stomach, intestines, liver, and pancreas.

**Gastroesophageal Junction** - The point where the esophagus meets the stomach, serving as a barrier to prevent reflux of stomach contents into the esophagus.

**Gastrointestinal Motility** - Refers to the movement of food and fluids through the digestive tract, facilitated by rhythmic contractions of the muscles lining the gastrointestinal system.

**Gastrointestinal Mucosa** - Refers to the inner lining of the digestive tract, consisting of epithelial cells, glands, and blood vessels, essential for nutrient absorption and protection against pathogens.

**Gastrointestinal Peristalsis** - The rhythmic contraction and relaxation of muscles in the digestive tract, facilitating the movement of food and fluids from the esophagus to the anus.

**Gastrointestinal Tract** - Also known as the digestive tract or alimentary canal, is the series of organs through which food and fluids pass, including the mouth, esophagus, stomach, intestines, and anus.

**Gastroparesis** - A condition characterized by delayed emptying of the stomach contents into the small intestine, leading to symptoms such as nausea, vomiting, and bloating.

**Gastroprokinetic Agent** - A medication that stimulates gastrointestinal motility, often used to treat conditions like gastroparesis and functional dyspepsia.

**Gaviscon** - An Antacid, over-the-counter medication used to relieve symptoms of heartburn, acid reflux, and indigestion by forming a protective barrier in the stomach. May Contain: Aluminum Hydroxide, Magnesium Carbonate and Sodium Alginate.

**Gaviscon Dual Action** - An Alginate, medication that provides fast relief from heartburn and indigestion by neutralizing stomach acid and forming a protective barrier to prevent acid reflux. May Contain: Sodium Alginate, Aluminum Hydroxide, and Magnesium Carbonate.

**General Anesthesia** - A state of controlled unconsciousness induced by medications to ensure pain relief, muscle relaxation, and loss of consciousness during surgical procedures.

**GER** - (or Gastroesophageal Reflux), which is the backward flow of stomach acid and contents into the esophagus, often causing heartburn and other symptoms.

**GERD** - Abbreviation for Gastroesophageal Reflux Disease, a chronic condition characterized by frequent episodes of acid reflux from the stomach into the esophagus, leading to symptoms such as heartburn and regurgitation.

**GFR** - (or Glomerular Filtration Rate), is a measure of kidney function that assesses the rate at which blood is filtered by the glomeruli per unit of time, reflecting kidney health.

**GI Motility** - Refers to the movement and coordination of muscles in the gastrointestinal tract, facilitating the digestion and propulsion of food through the stomach and intestines.

**GI Tract** - (or gastrointestinal tract), is the system of organs responsible for digestion and absorption of nutrients, including the mouth, esophagus, stomach, intestines, and anus.

**Ginger** - A root commonly used in cooking and traditional medicine, known for its anti-inflammatory and digestive properties, often used to alleviate nausea and gastrointestinal discomfort.

**Gingerols** - Bioactive compounds found in ginger, known for their anti-inflammatory and antioxidant properties, contributing to the health benefits associated with ginger consumption.

**Glandular Cells** - Specialized cells found in various organs and tissues that produce and secrete substances such as hormones, enzymes, or mucus, essential for normal physiological functions.

**Globus Pharyngeus** - A sensation of a lump or foreign body in the throat, often without an actual physical obstruction, commonly associated with stress or acid reflux.

**Glomerular Filtration Rate** - (or GFR), is a measure of kidney function that assesses the rate at which blood is filtered by the glomeruli per unit of time, reflecting kidney health.

**Glycyrrhiza Glabra** - The scientific name for licorice root, a herbaceous plant used in traditional medicine for its anti-inflammatory and expectorant properties.

**Glycyrrhizin** - A natural compound found in licorice root, known for its sweet taste and potential medicinal properties, but excessive consumption may lead to health issues like hypertension.

**Granulation** - The process of new tissue formation in wounds during the healing process, characterized by the growth of small, pinkish granules comprising blood vessels and fibroblasts.

**Gut Flora** - Refers to the diverse community of microorganisms, including bacteria, fungi, and viruses, residing in the digestive tract, essential for digestion, immune function, and overall health.

**Gut Microbiome** - Refers to the collection of microorganisms, including bacteria, viruses, and fungi, residing in the gastrointestinal tract, influencing various aspects of health and disease.

**Gut Microbiota** - Refers to the diverse community of microorganisms, including bacteria, fungi, and viruses, residing in the gastrointestinal tract, playing essential roles in digestion, immunity, and overall health.

**Gut-Associated Lymphoid Tissue** - (or GALT), is a component of the immune system located in the gastrointestinal tract, comprising lymphoid cells and structures that defend against pathogens and maintain immune balance.

**Gynecomastia** - The enlargement of breast tissue in males, often due to hormonal imbalances or medications, leading to breast swelling and tenderness.

# H

**H. Pylori Infections** - Bacterial infections of the stomach lining caused by Helicobacter pylori, often associated with gastritis, peptic ulcers, and increased risk of stomach cancer.

**H2 Blockers** - (or histamine-2 receptor antagonists), are a class of medications that inhibit the action of histamine on stomach cells, thereby reducing the production of gastric acid. They are commonly used to treat conditions like gastroesophageal reflux disease (GERD), peptic ulcers, and gastritis by alleviating symptoms such as heartburn, acid reflux, and stomach pain.

**H2 receptor Antagonists** - (or H2 blockers), are a class of medications that inhibit the action of histamine on stomach cells, thereby reducing the production of gastric acid. They are commonly used to treat conditions like gastroesophageal reflux.

**H2 Receptor Blockers** - Also known as histamine-2 receptor antagonists, are medications that alleviate symptoms of acid-related disorders by inhibiting histamine's action on stomach cells, thereby reducing the production of gastric acid. They are frequently prescribed for conditions like gastroesophageal reflux disease (GERD), peptic ulcers, and gastritis to relieve symptoms such as heartburn, acid reflux, and stomach pain.

**HCl** - (or Hydrochloric Acid), is a strong acid produced by the stomach that aids in digestion by breaking down food and killing bacteria.

**Heartburn** - A common symptom characterized by a burning sensation or discomfort in the chest, often accompanied by regurgitation of acidic stomach contents into the esophagus. It typically arises due to the reflux of stomach acid into the esophagus, resulting in irritation and inflammation of the esophageal lining.

**Helicobacter Pylori Bacterium** - A type of bacteria that infects the stomach lining, often leading to gastritis, peptic ulcers, and in some cases, stomach cancer.

**Hepatic Enzyme** - Proteins produced by the liver that play a crucial role in various metabolic processes, including detoxification, synthesis of proteins, and breakdown of nutrients.

**Hepatic Functions** - Refer to the essential roles performed by the liver in metabolism, detoxification, storage of nutrients, and synthesis of proteins and hormones.

**Hiatal Hernia** - A condition where a portion of the stomach protrudes into the chest cavity through the diaphragm, often causing symptoms such as heartburn and chest pain.

**Histamine** - A chemical compound released by the body's immune cells in response to injury, allergic reactions, or inflammation, playing a role in regulating various physiological processes such as allergic responses and gastric acid secretion.

**Holistic** - A holistic approach to healthcare takes into account not only physical symptoms but also mental, emotional, and spiritual aspects of a person's health and well-being. It views individuals as complex systems where all parts are interconnected and interdependent, recognizing that factors such as lifestyle, environment, emotions, and beliefs can influence overall health. This approach often involves personalized treatment plans that address the root causes of health issues rather than just managing symptoms, aiming to promote balance, harmony, and optimal health across all aspects of a person's life.

**Hydrochloric Acid** - (or HCl), is a strong acid produced by the stomach that aids in digestion by breaking down food and killing bacteria.

**Hydrogen-Potassium ATPase Enzyme System** - A cellular mechanism found in the stomach lining responsible for producing stomach acid, essential for digestion and killing ingested bacteria.

**Hyperacidity** - Refers to an excessive production of stomach acid, leading to symptoms such as heartburn, acid reflux, and stomach pain.

**Hypercalcemia** - A condition characterized by abnormally high levels of calcium in the blood, often causing symptoms such as excessive thirst, frequent urination, and abdominal pain.

**Hypermagnesemia** - A condition characterized by elevated levels of magnesium in the blood, potentially leading to symptoms such as muscle weakness, nausea, and cardiac abnormalities.

**Hypernatremia** - A condition characterized by elevated levels of sodium in the blood, often resulting from dehydration or excessive sodium intake, leading to symptoms such as thirst and altered mental status.

**Hypertension** - High blood pressure, a condition where the force of blood against the artery walls is consistently elevated, potentially leading to cardiovascular complications if left untreated.

# I

**IBS** - (or Irritable Bowel Syndrome), a chronic gastrointestinal disorder characterized by abdominal pain, bloating, and altered bowel habits, without evidence of structural abnormalities.

**Immunotherapy** - A treatment that enhances or modifies the body's immune system to recognize and destroy cancer cells or pathogens, often used in cancer and autoimmune disease treatments.

**Indigestion** - (or dyspepsia), is discomfort or pain in the upper abdomen, often accompanied by bloating, nausea, and heartburn, usually occurring after eating or drinking.

**Intestinal Motility** - Refers to the contraction and relaxation of muscles in the intestines, facilitating the movement of food and waste through the digestive tract.

**Ionic Forms** - Refer to chemical compounds or substances that exist as ions, either positively charged (cations) or negatively charged (anions), essential for various physiological processes in the body.

**Irritable Bowel Syndrome** - (or IBS), A chronic gastrointestinal disorder characterized by abdominal pain, bloating, and altered bowel habits, without evidence of structural abnormalities.

# K

**Kaopectate** - A Coating Agent class over-the-counter medication used to relieve diarrhea and upset stomach by coating the gastrointestinal tract and absorbing excess fluids. May Contain: Bismuth Subsalicylate

# L

**Lactose** - A sugar found in milk and dairy products that requires the enzyme lactase for proper digestion, intolerant individuals lack sufficient lactase enzyme.

**Lactose Intolerance** - The inability to digest lactose due to insufficient levels of the enzyme lactase, leading to gastrointestinal symptoms such as bloating, gas, and diarrhea after consuming dairy products.

**Lansoprazole** - A Proton Pump Inhibitor, medication used to reduce stomach acid production, treating conditions like gastroesophageal reflux disease (GERD), ulcers, and Zollinger-Ellison syndrome by alleviating symptoms and promoting healing (page 240).

**Laparoscopic Approach** - also known as minimally Invasive surgery, involves performing surgical procedures through small incisions using a camera and specialized instruments, resulting in less pain, quicker recovery, and minimal scarring.

**Laryngitis** - Inflammation of the larynx (voice box), often resulting in hoarseness, sore throat, and difficulty speaking, typically caused by viral infections or vocal strain.

**Laryngopharyngeal Reflux** - (or LPR) is the backward flow of stomach acid and contents into the throat and larynx, leading to symptoms such as hoarseness, throat clearing, and coughing.

**Laryngoscopy** - A procedure to examine the larynx (voice box) and nearby structures using a thin, flexible tube with a light and camera, often performed to diagnose conditions affecting the throat and vocal cords.

**Larynx** - (or voice box), is the organ in the throat responsible for producing sound and protecting the airway during swallowing, containing the vocal cords and facilitating speech.

**Laughter Yoga** - A practice combining laughter exercises and yogic breathing techniques to promote physical and emotional well-being through simulated laughter, group activities, and relaxation methods.

**Laxative** - Medications or substances that promote bowel movements, often used to relieve constipation by increasing stool frequency and softening stool consistency.

**Leptin** - A hormone produced by fat cells that regulates appetite and energy balance, signaling to the brain to reduce food intake and increase energy expenditure.

**LES** - (or Lower Esophageal Sphincter) is a circular muscle located at the junction of the esophagus and stomach, controlling the passage of food and preventing gastric reflux into the esophagus.

**Licorice** - A plant with sweet-tasting roots, used in traditional medicine for its potential health benefits, including soothing properties for gastrointestinal issues and sore throats.

**LINX Device** - A small, flexible ring made of magnetic beads surgically implanted around the lower esophageal sphincter (LES) to treat gastroesophageal reflux disease (GERD) by preventing acid reflux while preserving normal swallowing.

**Lipophilic (fat-soluble) Drugs** - Medications that dissolve easily in fat and are absorbed into fatty tissues, allowing them to be stored in the body for longer periods.

**Lower Esophageal Sphincter** - (or LES), is a circular muscle located at the junction of the esophagus and stomach, controlling the passage of food and preventing gastric reflux into the esophagus.

**LPR** - (or Laryngopharyngeal Reflux), is the backward flow of stomach acid and contents into the throat and larynx, leading to symptoms such as hoarseness, throat clearing, and coughing.

**Lycopene** - A natural pigment and antioxidant found in fruits and vegetables, particularly tomatoes, known for potential health benefits such as reducing the risk of certain cancers and protecting against heart disease.

# M

**Magnesium** - An essential mineral that plays a crucial role in various physiological functions, including muscle and nerve function, energy production, and bone health.

**Magnesium Chloride** - A dietary supplement or medication containing magnesium and chloride ions, often used to supplement magnesium levels in the body or as a treatment for magnesium deficiency.

**Magnesium Hydroxide** - An antacid medication used to neutralize stomach acid and provide relief from symptoms of heartburn, acid indigestion, and upset stomach (page 199, 280).

**Magnesium Stearate** - A commonly used pharmaceutical excipient, functioning as a lubricant in medication formulations to facilitate manufacturing and improve tablet or capsule disintegration.

**Malic Acid** - A natural substance found in various fruits and vegetables, often used as a food additive and supplement for its sour taste and potential health benefits.

**Marshmallow Root** - An herb derived from the Althaea Officinalis plant, used in traditional medicine for its soothing properties on the throat, digestive tract, and skin.

**Meditation** - A practice involving mindfulness or focused attention to promote relaxation, reduce stress, and enhance mental clarity and emotional well-being.

**Mechanism of Action -** The "mechanism of action" (MOA) refers to the specific biochemical interaction through which a drug substance produces its pharmacological effect. This term is crucial in pharmacology and medical science because understanding a drug's mechanism of action is key to comprehending how it works within the body to affect biological processes, treat a disease, or alleviate symptoms.

**Melatonin** - A hormone produced by the pineal gland that regulates sleep-wake cycles, often used as a supplement to treat sleep disorders.

**Metabolic Alkalosis** - A condition characterized by elevated blood pH and bicarbonate levels due to excess alkali intake, vomiting, or certain medical conditions, leading to symptoms such as muscle twitching and confusion.

**Metabolites** - Byproducts of metabolic processes in the body, including the breakdown of medications and nutrients, often measured in biological samples for diagnostic or research purposes.

**Metoclopramide** - A Prokinetic medication used to treat gastrointestinal disorders such as gastroparesis and acid reflux by increasing stomach contractions and reducing nausea and vomiting, often prescribed for short-term relief (page 257).

**Metoclopramide Hydrochloride** - A Prokinetic medication used to treat gastrointestinal disorders such as gastroparesis and acid reflux by promoting stomach contractions and relieving nausea and vomiting.

**Microbial Flora** - Refers to the diverse community of microorganisms, including bacteria, fungi, and viruses, residing in or on the body, playing essential roles in digestion, immunity, and overall health.

**Microbiome** - Refers to the collective genetic material and microorganisms, including bacteria, fungi, and viruses, residing in or on the body, influencing various aspects of health and disease.

**Microcrystalline Cellulose** - A commonly used pharmaceutical excipient derived from cellulose fibers, serving as a binder, filler, and disintegrant in medication formulations to improve tablet or capsule properties.

**Microorganisms** - Microscopic living organisms, including bacteria, viruses, fungi, and protozoa, often found in various environments, including the human body, and playing important roles in health and disease.

**Mindfulness** - A mental practice involving non-judgmental awareness of the present moment, often cultivated through meditation and exercises to reduce stress, enhance focus, and promote overall well-being.

**Monosodium Glutamate** - (or MSG), is a food additive used to enhance flavor, often found in processed foods, soups, and Asian cuisine, although some individuals may experience adverse reactions.

**Monounsaturated Fat** - Healthy dietary fats found in foods like olive oil, avocados, and nuts, associated with reducing bad cholesterol levels and lowering the risk of heart disease.

**Mosapride Citrate** - A Prokinetic medication used to treat gastrointestinal motility disorders such as gastroparesis and functional dyspepsia by enhancing stomach contractions and promoting gastric emptying (page 267).

**Motegrity** - A prokinetic, prescription medication for chronic idiopathic constipation in adults. It activates serotonin receptors in the gut to promote bowel movements, relieving constipation by increasing intestinal motility. May Contain: Prucalopride Succinate.

**Motility** - Refers to the movement and coordination of muscles in the gastrointestinal tract, facilitating the passage of food and waste materials through the digestive system.

**Motilium** - A prokinetic medication used to treat nausea, vomiting, and gastrointestinal motility disorders by blocking dopamine receptors in the digestive system, promoting normal movement and function. May Contain: Domperidone.

**MSG** - (or monosodium glutamate), is a food additive used to enhance flavor, often found in processed foods, soups, and Asian cuisine, although some individuals may experience adverse reactions.

**Mucilage** - A thick, gluey substance produced by certain plants, seeds, and microorganisms, often used in medicine for its soothing and protective properties on mucous membranes.

**Mylanta** - An Antacid, over-the-counter medication, used to relieve symptoms of heartburn, acid indigestion, and gas by neutralizing stomach acid and breaking up gas bubbles in the stomach. May Contain: Aluminum Hydroxide, Magnesium Hydroxide and Simethicone.

# N

**Nasopharynx** - The upper part of the throat located behind the nose, connecting the nasal cavity to the upper part of the throat and serving as a passage for air and drainage of mucus.

**Nei-Kuan (P6) Point** - An acupressure point located on the inner wrist, commonly used in traditional Chinese medicine to relieve nausea, vomiting, and motion sickness.

**Nexium** - A proton pump inhibitor, medication used to treat conditions like gastroesophageal reflux disease (GERD) and ulcers by reducing stomach acid production. May Contain: Esomeprazole.

**Nissen Fundoplication** - A surgical procedure to treat gastroesophageal reflux disease (GERD) by wrapping the upper part of the stomach around the lower esophagus to strengthen the lower esophageal sphincter and prevent acid reflux.

**Nizatidine** - An H2 Blocker, medication used to treat conditions like ulcers and gastroesophageal reflux disease (GERD) by reducing stomach acid production (page 221).

**Non-Heme Iron** - A type of dietary iron found in plant-based foods and fortified products, less easily absorbed by the body compared to heme iron found in animal sources.

**Non-Steroidal Anti-Inflammatory Drugs** (or NSAIDs) - Medications used to reduce inflammation, pain, and fever by inhibiting prostaglandin production, commonly used for conditions like arthritis and minor aches.

**NSAIDs** - (or Non-steroidal anti-inflammatory drugs), are medications used to reduce inflammation, pain, and fever by inhibiting prostaglandin production, commonly used for conditions like arthritis and minor aches.

**Nutrient Malabsorption** - Refers to the impaired absorption of nutrients in the digestive tract, leading to deficiencies and health problems due to conditions like celiac disease or gastrointestinal surgery.

# O

**Obesity** - A medical condition characterized by excess body fat accumulation, often resulting from a combination of genetic, environmental, and lifestyle factors, increasing the risk of various health problems.

**Odynophagia** - The medical term for painful swallowing, often caused by inflammation or injury to the throat, esophagus, or nearby structures, leading to discomfort during swallowing.

**Omeprazole** - A proton pump inhibitor, medication that works by blocking the enzyme responsible for acid production in the stomach, providing relief from symptoms such as heartburn, acid indigestion, and gastroesophageal reflux disease (GERD) (page 234).

**Oral Microbiome** - Refers to the diverse community of microorganisms, including bacteria, fungi, and viruses, residing in the mouth, influencing oral health and contributing to various conditions such as dental caries and gum disease.

**Osteoporosis** - A medical condition characterized by weakening and thinning of bones, increasing the risk of fractures, often associated with aging, hormonal changes, and nutritional deficiencies.

**Oxidative Stress** - An imbalance between the production of reactive oxygen species (free radicals) and the body's ability to detoxify them, leading to cellular damage and contributing to various diseases.

**Oxygen Therapy** - A medical treatment involving the administration of supplemental oxygen used to increase oxygen levels in the blood, commonly delivered via nasal cannula, face mask, or ventilator, to treat conditions such as respiratory failure, pneumonia, and chronic obstructive pulmonary disease (COPD).

# P

**Pancreas** - A glandular organ located behind the stomach, producing digestive enzymes and insulin to regulate blood sugar levels, essential for digestion and metabolism.

**Pantoprazole** - A proton pump inhibitor medication that works by inhibiting the enzyme responsible for acid production in the stomach, providing relief from symptoms such as heartburn, acid indigestion, and gastroesophageal reflux disease (GERD) (page 243).

**Paraesophageal** - Refers to anatomical structures or conditions located adjacent to or surrounding the esophagus, often used to describe hernias or abnormalities involving tissues near the esophagus.

**Parasympathetic Nervous System** - A division of the autonomic nervous system responsible for controlling involuntary bodily functions, promoting relaxation, digestion, and conservation of energy.

**Parietal Cells** - Specialized cells found in the lining of the stomach that secrete hydrochloric acid and intrinsic factor, playing a crucial role in digestion and nutrient absorption, particularly vitamin B12.

**Pathogenic Bacteria** - Microorganisms capable of causing disease in the host organism by invading tissues, producing toxins, or triggering inflammatory responses, leading to illness and infection.

**Pathogens** - Microorganisms, such as bacteria, viruses, fungi, or parasites, capable of causing disease in their host organisms by infecting tissues, disrupting normal bodily functions, and triggering immune responses.

**Pectin** - A soluble fiber found in fruits, used in medicine and food as a thickening agent and to promote digestive health by aiding in bowel regularity and lowering cholesterol levels.

**Pepcid AC** - An H2 Blocker, over-the-counter medication used to relieve heartburn, acid indigestion, and sour stomach by reducing stomach acid production. May Contain: Famotidine

**Pepsin** - A digestive enzyme produced in the stomach, primarily responsible for breaking down proteins into smaller peptides for absorption, aiding in the digestion of dietary proteins into amino acids.

**Pepsinogen** - An inactive precursor enzyme secreted by the stomach's chief cells, which is activated by stomach acid to form pepsin, playing a key role in protein digestion in the stomach.

**Peptac** - An Alginate, over-the-counter medication, used to relieve symptoms of heartburn and acid reflux by forming a protective barrier in the stomach. May Contain: Sodium Alginate, Sodium Bicarbonate, and Calcium Carbonate.

**Peptic Ulcers** - Open sores or lesions that develop in the lining of the stomach, small intestine, or esophagus due to erosion from stomach acid or infection with Helicobacter pylori bacteria.

**Peptides** - Short chains of amino acids, the building blocks of proteins, involved in various physiological functions and signaling pathways within the body, often with specific biological activities.

**Pepto-Bismol** - A coating Agent, over-the-counter medication containing bismuth subsalicylate. Used to relieve symptoms of indigestion, upset stomach, and diarrhea by coating the stomach lining and reducing inflammation. May Contain: Bismuth Subsalicylate.

**Peristalsis** - The coordinated muscle contractions that propel food and fluids through the digestive tract, facilitating digestion and absorption by moving contents along the gastrointestinal tract in a wave-like manner.

**Peristaltic Reflex** - An automatic, coordinated contraction and relaxation of muscles in the digestive tract, initiated by the stretching of the gastrointestinal wall, facilitating the movement of food and fluids through the digestive system.

**PET Scans** - (or Positron Emission Tomography Scans), are imaging tests that use radioactive tracers to detect cellular activity and metabolic processes within the body, aiding in the diagnosis and monitoring of various medical conditions.

**PH Level** - Measures the acidity or alkalinity of a substance, indicating its concentration of hydrogen ions. It's crucial for maintaining the body's physiological balance and proper function of biological processes.

**Pharmacodynamics** - Refers to how drugs interact with the body to produce their effects, encompassing mechanisms of action, drug-receptor interactions, and physiological responses to medications.

**Pharmacokinetics** - The study of how drugs are absorbed, distributed, metabolized, and excreted by the body, influencing the drug's concentration and duration of action within the body.

**Phosphate Binder** - A medication used to lower phosphate levels in the blood by binding to dietary phosphate in the gastrointestinal tract, often prescribed for individuals with kidney disease.

**Phosphate Levels** - Refer to the concentration of phosphate ions in the blood, essential for various biological processes such as bone formation, energy metabolism, and cell signaling.

**Pilates** - A form of exercise that focuses on strengthening muscles, improving flexibility, and enhancing body awareness through controlled movements and breathing techniques, often practiced for fitness and rehabilitation.

**Placebo Effect** - Refers to the phenomenon where a patient's condition improves after receiving an inert substance or sham treatment, solely due to their belief in the treatment's effectiveness.

**Polymorphisms** - Variations in DNA sequence among individuals, affecting genes' structure or function, potentially influencing susceptibility to diseases, drug responses, and other biological traits.

**Polypharmacy** - The use of multiple medications by a patient, often involving the concurrent use of several drugs to manage multiple health conditions, potentially increasing the risk of adverse drug reactions and interactions.

**Polysaccharide** - A complex carbohydrate composed of long chains of sugar molecules, serving as energy storage molecules in plants and structural components in organisms such as cellulose and glycogen.

**Polysaccharides** - Complex carbohydrates consisting of multiple sugar molecules bonded together, serving various functions in the body, including energy storage, structural support, and cell signaling.

**Polyunsaturated Fats** - Healthy dietary fats found in plant-based oils, seeds, and fatty fish, containing multiple double bonds in their chemical structure and beneficial for heart health when consumed in moderation.

**Postprandial Heartburn** - A burning sensation in the chest or throat that occurs after eating, often due to stomach acid refluxing into the esophagus, causing discomfort or pain.

**PPIs** - (or Proton Pump Inhibitors), are medications that block the proton pump enzyme in the stomach lining, reducing acid production and providing relief from conditions like acid reflux, ulcers, and GERD.

**Pranayama** - Yoga practice involving breath control techniques aimed at regulating and enhancing the flow of vital energy (prana) within the body, promoting physical, mental, and spiritual well-being.

**Prevacid** - A proton pump inhibitor, used to treat conditions like acid reflux, ulcers, and GERD by reducing stomach acid production and providing relief from associated symptoms. May Contain: Lansoprazole.

**Prilosec** - A proton pump inhibitor, used to treat conditions like acid reflux, ulcers, and GERD by reducing stomach acid production and providing relief from associated symptoms. May Contain: Omeprazole.

**Probiotics** - Live microorganisms, such as bacteria and yeast, that provide health benefits when consumed in adequate amounts, supporting digestive health and immune function by restoring the balance of beneficial gut bacteria.

**Progesterone** - A hormone produced by the ovaries (in women), adrenal glands, and placenta (during pregnancy), playing a key role in regulating the menstrual cycle, supporting pregnancy, and maintaining reproductive health.

**Progressive Muscle Relaxation** - (or PMR), a technique involving the systematic tensing and relaxing of muscle groups throughout the body, used to reduce stress, alleviate muscle tension, and promote relaxation.

**Prokinetics** - Medications that enhance gastrointestinal motility by stimulating muscle contractions in the digestive tract, aiding in the movement of food and fluids through the stomach and intestines. They're used to treat conditions like gastroparesis.

**Prolactin** - A hormone secreted by the pituitary gland that plays a role in lactation, breast development, and reproductive function, primarily in females but also present in males at lower levels.

**Prostaglandins** - Lipid compounds produced in various tissues throughout the body, acting as signaling molecules to regulate inflammation, smooth muscle contraction, blood clotting, and other physiological processes.

**Proton Pump Inhibitors** - (or PPIs), Medications that block the proton pump enzyme in the stomach lining, reducing acid production and providing relief from conditions like acid reflux, ulcers, and GERD.

**Protonix** - A proton pump inhibitor medication used to treat conditions like acid reflux, ulcers, and GERD by reducing stomach acid production and providing relief from associated symptoms. May Contain: Pantoprazole.

**Prucalopride Succinate** - A Prokinetic medication used to treat chronic constipation by enhancing gastrointestinal motility, specifically by activating serotonin receptors in the gut to stimulate bowel movements (page 264).

**Pyrosis** - Medical term commonly known as heartburn, is a burning sensation in the chest caused by the reflux of stomach acid into the esophagus, often occurring after eating or when lying down.

# Q

**Qi** - In traditional Chinese medicine, refers to vital energy or life force that flows through the body, influencing health and well-being. It is believed to regulate bodily functions and maintain balance within the body.

**QT Interval Prolongation** - A cardiac condition characterized by lengthening of the time it takes for the heart's electrical system to repolarize, potentially leading to dangerous arrhythmias and sudden cardiac death.

# R

**Rabeprazole** - A proton pump inhibitor medication, used to treat conditions like acid reflux, ulcers, and GERD by reducing stomach acid production and providing relief from associated symptoms (page 246).

**Radiation Therapy** - A cancer treatment that uses high-energy radiation to destroy cancer cells or shrink tumors, often used alone or in combination with other treatments like surgery or chemotherapy.

**Radiofrequency Ablation** - (or RFA), a minimally invasive procedure that uses heat generated from high-frequency radio waves to destroy abnormal tissues, such as tumors or abnormal heart rhythm sites, while minimizing damage to surrounding healthy tissues.

**Reflexologist** - A practitioner who applies pressure to specific points on the hands, feet, or ears believed to correspond to various organs and systems in the body, aiming to promote relaxation and improve overall health.

**Reflexology** - A complementary therapy that involves applying pressure to specific points on the hands, feet, or ears to stimulate relaxation, relieve tension, and promote healing in corresponding organs and systems of the body.

**Reglan** - A prokinetic medication that enhances gastrointestinal motility and aids in gastric emptying by increasing muscle contractions in the digestive tract, commonly used to treat conditions like gastroparesis and acid reflux. May Contain: Metoclopramide Hydrochloride.

**Relaxin** - A hormone primarily secreted by the ovaries and placenta during pregnancy, which helps to soften connective tissues, relax pelvic ligaments, and facilitate childbirth by widening the birth canal.

**Renal Functions** - Refers to the kidneys' ability to filter waste products from the blood, regulate fluid balance, maintain electrolyte concentrations, and produce hormones critical for blood pressure regulation and red blood cell production.

**Reye's Syndrome** - A rare but serious condition primarily affecting children and teenagers, characterized by acute brain and liver inflammation, often occurring after viral infections and associated with aspirin use.

**RFA** - (or Radiofrequency Ablation), a minimally invasive procedure that uses heat generated from high-frequency radio waves to destroy abnormal tissues, such as tumors or abnormal heart rhythm sites, while minimizing damage to surrounding healthy tissues.

**Rolaids** - An Antacid, over-the-counter antacid medication, used to neutralize stomach acid and provide relief from symptoms of indigestion, heartburn, and upset stomach. May Contain: Calcium Carbonate and Magnesium Hydroxide.

**Rolling Hiatal Hernia** - Occurs when the stomach protrudes into the chest through the diaphragm, potentially causing symptoms like heartburn, chest pain, and difficulty swallowing.

# S

**S-isomer of Omeprazole** - Refers to a specific configuration of a molecule, often denoting a particular form or variant of a compound.

**Salicylate Content** - Refers to the concentration of salicylic acid or its derivatives in a substance, often associated with medications like aspirin or topical products used for their anti-inflammatory, analgesic, or antipyretic properties.

**Secretin** - A hormone produced in the small intestine that stimulates the pancreas to release bicarbonate-rich fluids, aiding in neutralizing stomach acid and promoting digestion in the small intestine.

**Serotonin (5-HT4) Receptor Agonist** - A medication that activates serotonin receptors in the gastrointestinal tract, promoting gastrointestinal motility and enhancing bowel movements, commonly used to treat conditions like chronic constipation or irritable bowel syndrome with constipation.

**Serotonin Receptors** - Proteins located on cell membranes throughout the body, including the brain and gastrointestinal tract, that bind to serotonin neurotransmitters, influencing various physiological functions such as mood regulation, appetite, sleep, and gastrointestinal motility.

**Serum Phosphate Levels** - Refer to the concentration of phosphate ions in the blood, which play a crucial role in bone health, energy metabolism, and cellular function, and are regulated by hormonal and renal mechanisms.

**Serum Prolactin** - Refers to the level of the hormone prolactin present in the blood, which regulates lactation, reproductive function, and various other physiological processes, with abnormal levels potentially indicating underlying health conditions.

**Silent Reflux** - Also known as laryngopharyngeal reflux (LPR), is a condition where stomach acid flows back into the throat and larynx without causing typical symptoms of heartburn, often leading to throat irritation, hoarseness, coughing, or difficulty swallowing.

**Simethicone** - An Antacid, over-the-counter medication used to relieve symptoms of gas and bloating by breaking up gas bubbles in the digestive tract, facilitating their elimination and providing relief from discomfort (page 207).

**Sliding Hiatal Hernia** - Occurs when the stomach and part of the esophagus slide up into the chest through the diaphragm, potentially causing symptoms like heartburn, regurgitation, and chest pain.

**Sodium Alginate** - A natural substance derived from seaweed used in medications and dietary supplements for its ability to form a protective barrier in the stomach, providing relief from acid reflux and heartburn (page 274).

**Sodium Bicarbonate** - Also known as baking soda, is a chemical compound used as an antacid to neutralize excess stomach acid and alleviate symptoms of indigestion, heartburn, and upset stomach (page 205, 283).

**Sodium Ions** - Positively charged particles found in bodily fluids, playing essential roles in regulating fluid balance, nerve function, muscle contraction, and maintaining cellular integrity and electrical gradients.

**Sodium Starch Glycolate** - A pharmaceutical excipient used in tablet formulations to aid in disintegration, allowing tablets to dissolve quickly and release their active ingredients for absorption in the gastrointestinal tract.

**Somnolence** - A state of drowsiness or sleepiness, often characterized by a strong desire to sleep or difficulty staying awake, which can be caused by various factors including medications, illness, or fatigue.

**Spleen Meridians** - Refer to energy pathways in traditional Chinese medicine believed to be associated with the spleen organ, influencing physiological functions, emotions, and overall health when balanced or disrupted.

**Squamous Cell Carcinoma** - A type of skin cancer that arises from squamous cells in the outermost layer of the skin, typically developing on sun-exposed areas and characterized by scaly, red patches or nodules.

**Squamous Epithelium** - A type of epithelial tissue characterized by flattened, scale-like cells arranged in layers, found in the skin, respiratory tract, and lining of certain organs, providing protection and facilitating diffusion.

**Stomach Acid** - Or gastric acid, is a digestive fluid produced by the stomach's parietal cells, primarily composed of hydrochloric acid (HCl), essential for breaking down food, sterilizing the stomach, and aiding in nutrient absorption.

**Stomach Strangulation** - A medical emergency where the blood supply to the stomach is cut off, typically due to twisting or obstruction of the stomach, leading to tissue damage and potential organ failure.

**Subluxation** - Partial dislocations of a joint where the bones are misaligned but still in contact, potentially causing pain, restricted movement, and neurological dysfunction, often treated by chiropractors.

**Swedish Bitters** - A herbal remedy composed of a blend of bitter-tasting herbs such as aloe, myrrh, and angelica root, traditionally believed to promote digestion, stimulate appetite, and support overall health and wellness when taken in small doses.

**Synthetic Medications** - Pharmaceutical drugs formulated through chemical synthesis rather than derived from natural sources, designed to mimic or enhance the effects of naturally occurring compounds for therapeutic purposes.

# T

**Tagamet HB** - An H2 Blocker, over-the-counter medication used to relieve symptoms of heartburn and acid indigestion by reducing stomach acid production and providing relief from gastric discomfort. May Contain: Cimetidine.

**Tardive Dyskinesia** - A neurological disorder characterized by involuntary and repetitive movements, often affecting the face, tongue, or limbs, caused by long-term use of certain medications, especially antipsychotic drugs.

**Targeted Therapy** - A cancer treatment approach that uses drugs or other substances to specifically identify and attack cancer cells, often by targeting specific molecules or pathways involved in the growth and survival of cancer cells.

**Tarry Stools** - Also known as melena, are dark, sticky stools caused by the presence of digested blood in the stool, often indicating bleeding in the upper gastrointestinal tract, such as the stomach or esophagus.

**Terpenoids** - A diverse class of organic compounds found in plants and some insects, characterized by their structure based on units of isoprene, often possessing aromatic or medicinal properties and serving various biological functions.

**Tetracycline Antibiotics** - A group of broad-spectrum antibiotics that inhibit bacterial protein synthesis, commonly used to treat various bacterial infections such as acne, respiratory tract infections, and sexually transmitted diseases.

**Tooth Enamel** - The hard, outermost layer of the tooth structure, primarily composed of minerals like hydroxyapatite, providing protection against decay and mechanical wear while maintaining tooth shape and color.

**Toupet Fundoplication** - A surgical procedure used to treat gastroesophageal reflux disease (GERD) by wrapping the fundus of the stomach around the lower esophagus, reinforcing the lower esophageal sphincter and reducing acid reflux.

**Tricyclic Antidepressant Overdose** - Refers to the ingestion of excessive amounts of tricyclic antidepressant medications, leading to toxic effects such as cardiac arrhythmias, seizures, coma, and potentially fatal outcomes.

**Tums** - An Antacid, over-the-counter antacid medication used to relieve symptoms of heartburn, acid indigestion, and upset stomach by neutralizing excess stomach acid and providing temporary relief. May Contain: Calcium Carbonate.

# U

**UES** - (or Upper Esophageal Sphincter), a muscular valve at the upper end of the esophagus, regulating the passage of food and fluids from the pharynx into the esophagus during swallowing and preventing air from entering.

**Ulmus Rubra Tree** - Commonly known as the slippery elm tree, is a deciduous tree native to North America, traditionally used in herbal medicine for its mucilaginous bark, which is believed to have soothing and anti-inflammatory properties.

**Upper Esophageal Sphincter** - (or UES), a muscular valve at the upper end of the esophagus, regulating the passage of food and fluids from the pharynx into the esophagus during swallowing and preventing air from entering.

# V

**Vagus Nerve** - The tenth cranial nerve, playing a crucial role in regulating various bodily functions, including digestion, heart rate, respiratory rate, and many aspects of the parasympathetic nervous system.

**Virtual Reality** - (or VR), is a computer-generated simulation of a three-dimensional environment, allowing users to interact with and experience artificial sensory stimuli, often used for entertainment, training, therapy, and medical applications.

# Y

**Yoga** - A mind-body practice originating from ancient India, involving physical postures, breathing exercises, and meditation techniques, aimed at promoting physical and mental well-being, flexibility, strength, and relaxation.

**Yoga - Ardha Matsyendrasana** (Half Spinal Twist) - A yoga pose that involves twisting the spine while seated, providing stretching benefits for the back, shoulders, and hips, as well as stimulating digestion and detoxification.

**Yoga - Marjariasana** (Cat-Cow Stretch) - A yoga pose that involves arching and rounding the spine alternately, promoting flexibility and mobility in the spine, and gently stretching the back and abdominal muscles.

**Yoga - Uttana Shishosana** (Extended Puppy Pose) - A yoga pose that involves stretching the spine and shoulders while resting the hips high, promoting flexibility in the spine, shoulders, and arms, and relieving tension.

**Yoga - Vajrasana** (Thunderbolt Pose) - A yoga pose that involves sitting on the heels with the spine straight, promoting digestion, relieving back and knee pain, and improving posture.

# Z

**Zantac 360°** - An H2 Blocker, over-the-counter medication used to treat heartburn and acid indigestion by reducing stomach acid production for extended relief. May Contain: Famotidine.

**Zinc Carnosine** - A supplement compound composed of zinc and L-carnosine, used to support gastrointestinal health, promote healing of the stomach lining, and protect against gastric ulcers and other digestive issues.

**Zollinger-Ellison Syndrome** - A rare disorder characterized by excessive production of stomach acid, leading to peptic ulcers, severe abdominal pain, diarrhea, and other digestive complications due to gastrin-secreting tumors in the pancreas or duodenum.

# ♡ Thank You ♡

I'm thrilled at the prospect that this book has not only lifted your spirits and sparked inspiration within you but has also equipped you with actionable strategies to step into a life brimming with health and vitality. I envision many of you seizing the power to free yourselves from the shackles of medication, or at the very least, significantly reducing your dependence on them.

Additionally, by investigating the details of various medications, my aim was to enhance your understanding of the treatments you have been relying on, thereby enabling you to make empowered, well-informed decisions about your health as you move forward.

As we conclude, If you've found value in these pages, I would sincerely appreciate your taking a moment to leave a positive review wherever you discovered this book. I will be reading each and every comment, with each being a tremendous source of encouragement for me.

Thank you for your support, and for joining me on this journey.

With Heartfelt Gratitude... Lillian Heart ♡